AF385718

Recent Results in Cancer Research

85

Fortschritte der Krebsforschung
Progrès dans les recherches sur le cancer

Editor in Chief: P. Rentchnik, Genève
Co-editor: H. J. Senn, St. Gallen

Urologic Cancer: Chemotherapeutic Principles and Management

Edited by Frank M. Torti

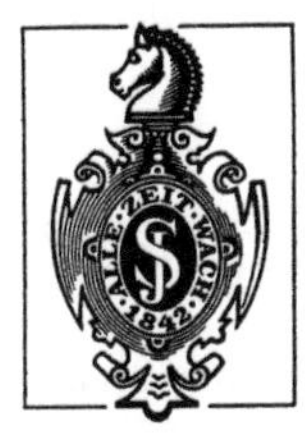

Springer-Verlag
Berlin Heidelberg New York Tokyo 1983

Frank M. Torti, MD

Division of Medical Oncology
Stanford University Medical Center
Palo Alto Veterans Administration Medical Center
and the Northern California Cancer Program
Palo Alto, CA, USA

Sponsored by the Swiss League against Cancer

ISBN-13:978-3-642-81996-4   e-ISBN-13:978-3-642-81994-0
DOI: 10.1007/978-3-642-81994-0

Library of Congress Cataloging in Publication Data. Main entry under title: Urologic Cancer: Chemotherapeutic Principles and Management. (Recent results in cancer research; 85) Bibliography: p. Includes index. 1. Urinary organs–Cancer–Chemotherapy. 2. Antineoplastic agents. I. Torti, F. M. (Frank M.), 1947-. II. Series. [DNLM: 1. Urologic neoplasms–Drug therapy. W1 RE106P v. 85/WJ 160 C5175] RC261.R35 vol. 85 [RC280.U74] 616.99′4s 82-25600 [616.99′462061]

2125/3140–543210

For Dorothea, Frankie, Suzy and T.

Contents

List of Contributors

S. K. Carter
Northern California Cancer Program, P.O. Box 10144,
Palo Alto, CA 94303, USA

W. G. Harker
Division of Medical Oncology, Department of Medicine,
Stanford University Medical Center, Stanford, CA 94305, USA

B. L. Lum
Clinical Research Pharmacist, Northern California Oncology
Group, Palo Alto, CA, USA

F. J. Meyers
Division of Hematology/Oncology, University of California,
Davis Medical Center, Sacramento, Ca, USA

F. M. Torti
Division of Medical Oncology, Stanford University Medical
Center, Palo Alto, Ca, USA

Introduction: The Multidisciplinary Approach to the Treatment of Urologic Malignancy

F. M. Torti

Division of Medical Oncology, Stanford University Medical Center, Palo Alto, CA, USA

Progress in the treatment of patients with cancers of the uroepithelium has been the result of both technologic and conceptual advances. Computerized tomographic scans, intensive post-operative management, radiation implants, and other technologic advances have been combined with a better understanding of phenomena such as downstaging in bladder cancer and the biologic variability of prostate cancer. This progress has been nourished by the longstanding multidisciplinary effort of surgeons and radiation therapists. This interaction has led to a better definition of the uses and limitations of each discipline in cancer of the testis, prostate, penis, bladder, and kidney. Recent advances in chemotherapy have lead to the integration of the medical oncologist into this multidisciplinary effort.

Urologic cancer is a microcosm of the entire spectrum of the efficacy of chemotherapy in malignant disease. In testicular carcinoma, patients with advanced disease can be cured in more than half of cases with chemotherapy alone or in combination with surgery. In bladder cancer, although there are few if any durable complete responses, many patients with advanced symptomatic disease can be effectively palliated. Prostatic carcinoma is also a disease where chemotherapy can be palliative, although not to the degree or with the frequency of metastatic bladder cancer. Carcinoma of the penis is a rare malignancy in which the definition of the exact role and utility of chemotherapy has been limited by the rarity of the disease in our population. Renal cell carcinoma remains almost entirely refractory to therapy once the disease has extended beyond surgical cure.

Like any new treatment, the incorporation of chemotherapy into the treatment planning in patients with urologic malignancies redefines an entire range of surgical, radiation, and hormonal treatments in relation to the chemotherapeutic approach. For example, the success of chemotherapy in testicular cancer in advanced disease has forced a reexploration of the role of chemotherapy as a surgical adjuvant in early stage testicular cancer. In bladder cancer, as well, trials of adjuvant chemotherapy are now underway. Even in the treatment of superficial bladder cancer, the role and timing of surgery is being rethought in relation to the currently effective intravesical agents. Thus, although the major emphasis of this book is on the chemotherapy of urologic cancers, this can only be addressed effectively in the context of the overall therapeutic strategy for each disease. Each of the authors has, therefore, integrated the chemotherapeutic data into the framework of the overall disease treatment. In testicular carcinoma, for example, Dr. Carter has approached the disease even in its early stages since chemotherapy continues to be discussed and tested earlier in testicular cancer. In the chapter on penile carcinoma, Dr. Meyers has emphasized the limited data and therefore the difficulty in defining the appropriate role for

Recent Results in Cancer Research. Vol. 85
© Springer-Verlag Berlin · Heidelberg 1983

chemotherapy. In the prostatic carcinoma, an entire chapter has been devoted to response criteria, which are critical to any discussion of chemotherapeutic efficacy. In renal cell cancer, chemotherapy has been related to other approaches to metastatic diseases, including surgical an hormonal treatment.

The spectrum of neoplasia seen in the urogenital tract represents a broad range of disease with challenging and variable natural histories which have taxed the ingenuity of physicians for many years. It is hoped that this comprehensive review of the chemotherapy of urologic cancer will aid the physician in the increasingly complex treatment decisions that must be made for optimal patient management.

Intravesical Chemotherapy of Superficial Bladder Cancer

B. L. Lum

Northern California Oncology Group, Palo Alto, CA, USA

Introduction

Bladder cancer accounts for 4.4% of the new cases of cancer diagnosed each year in the United States. It was estimated in 1982 that 37,100 new cases of bladder cancer would be seen, with 27,000 cases appearing in males and 10,100 in females [4]. This sex-related dominance is probably a reflection of the preponderance of industrial exposure to chemical carcinogens and cigarette smoking in the male population [21, 22, 25, 85, 92, 106, 169]. These statistics do not include carcinoma in situ. It was also estimated in 1982 that 10,600 deaths would result from bladder cancer [4]. This is a 6% increase in the incidence of bladder cancer and a 3% increase in bladder cancer deaths from 1980 estimates [5]. Histologically, these tumors arise from the bladder epithelium, with transitional cell carcinoma accounting for approximately 90% of the cases, squamous cell carcinomas for 8%, and adenocarcinomas for the remaining 2% [129]. Of these newly diagnosed cases, 75%−85% of patients initially present with superficial (localized) tumors [5]; that is, tumors which would fall into the Jewett-Strong-Marshall classification of stage 0 or A tumors and would be classified at pathologic stage Pa, PIS, or P1 in the TNM system [76, 99, 141, 172] (Table 1). These tumors either show no evidence of invasion (0) or invasion of the lamina propria but not the superficial muscle (A). This includes the group of patients with carcinoma in

Table 1. Staging for bladder cancer

Extent of disease	Jewett-Strong-Marshall	UICC (T or P)
Carcinoma in situ	0	Tis, No, Mo
Papilloma	0	Ta, No, Mo
Invasion not beyond lamina propria	A	T1, No, Mo
Invasion into superficial muscle	B1	T2, No, Mo
Invasion into deep muscle	B2	T3, No, Mo
Invasion into perivesical fat	C	T3, No, Mo
Invasion into adjacent organs or Invasion into regional lymph nodes	D1	T4, N±
Invasion into extrapelvic lymph nodes or Distant metastasis	D2	T4, N+M±

T, clinical stage; *P*, pathologic stage; *D1*, lymph node metastasis below level of the aortic bifurcation; *D2*, lymph node metastasis above the level of the aortic bifurcation

Recent Results in Cancer Research. Vol. 85
© Springer-Verlag Berlin · Heidelberg 1983

situ. Of the remaining patients, 10% are found to have regional (infiltrative) disease and 5% present with distant disease. Because of the preponderance of transitional cell carcinoma in cancers of the bladder and the poor prognosis for patients with squamous cell carcinomas of the bladder, or adenocarcinomas of the bladder, subsequent discussion will be limited to the transitional cell type [2, 55, 72, 77, 140, 188].

Factors That Influence the Natural and Therapeutic History of Superficial Bladder Cancer

The natural and therapeutic histories of the bladder tumors overlap. There are no purely observational series reported in the literature; however, the natural history of the disease may be judged to some extent through the surgical series [187], which have been described extensively in the literature, and to some extent, through the literature concerning intravesival chemotherapy. It is important to realize that these tumors constitute a spectrum of tumors with disparate biologic behavior and dissimilar survival rates. Overall, if one examines the 5-year survival of patients with superficial bladder cancers treated with transurethral resection (TUR) alone, one observes 5-year survival rates of approximately 70% in patients with clinical stage 0 tumors [30], 43%−77% in patients with stage A disease [9, 30, 51, 98, 107, 128], and approximately 60% in patients with stage B1 neoplasms [9, 107, 128]. One must keep in mind that these series are quite heterogeneous as far as the influence of the other factors mentioned below that influence survival. This data, approximate as it may be, does express that these tumors, although confined to the category of superficial tumors of the bladder mucosa, do have a small but measurable potential for causing cancer-related deaths. Any attempt to unterstand the natural and therapeutic history of superficial bladder tumors must take into account categorizations of the tumor other than clinical stage. These include factors such as grade, multicentricity (polychrono-topicity), the variable nature of carcinoma in situ, as well as other factors related to new occurrences, such as tumor implantation.
The incidence of tumor recurrence following initial therapy for superficial bladder tumors ranges from 40% to 85% [3, 8, 55, 91, 93, 140, 143, 173, 188]. Most occur within 6−12 months. This variation in reported recurrence rates is probably a reflection of the factors mentioned above. Utz and associates [173] reported an 82% recurrence rate within 1 year of initial therapy in 62 patients with carcinoma in situ of the bladder. Lerman ét al. [91] revealed an overall recurrence rate of 47% in patients with bladder papillomas. However, it was noted that that if the initial lesions was unifocal, there was recurrence in only 31% of the patients, wereas if the initial presentation was one of multiple papillomas, the recurrence rate was 66%. In contrast, Loening and associates found an overall 12 month recurrence rate of 57% in 153 follow-up patients. These investigators reported that the initial size, grade, or number of tumors did not significantly influence the 12-month recurrence. Of the study patients recurring, 85% did so within 12 months of study entry [93]. Some recurrences have been noted to occur at a higher stage and/or grade and may recur temporally and spatially as multiple tumors [3, 91, 143, 179]. Since the vast majority of patients who develop superficial bladder cancer do so between the ages of 50−70 years of age [33], survival is often a difficult endpoint in the evaluation of these patients, since deaths due to current illness make up a substantial portion of any survival. Failure of the local treatment of superficial bladder cancer may be best defined by the development of

Table 2. Recurrence, invasion, and survival in superficial bladder cancer

Author	Number of patients	Stage reported	Recurrence %	Invasion %	5-year survival %	Mean time to invasion	Reference no.
Denning 1950	109	Ta	69	7.3	—	—	[34]
Nichols and Marshall 1956	86	T1	—	—	84	—	[122]
Pyrah et al. 1964	207	Ta	54	6.6	—	—	[143]
Lerman et al. 1970	125	Ta	66 (M) 31 (S)	9.5	88	7.6 years	[91]
Greene et al. 1973	100	T1	73	10.0	80	—	[55]
O'Flynn et al. 1975	126	T1	—	—	62	—	[128]
Althausen et al. 1976	129	TIS, Atypia	85	30[a]	100	3 years	[3]
Williams et al. 1977	167	T1	50	7.8	72	3–5 years	[188]
Barnes et al. 1977	64	A	—	—	73	—	[9]
MacKenzie et al. 1981	292	0–B1	53	25	—	18 months	[96]
Lutzeyer et al. 1982	315	Ta–T2	64	—	97 (Ta Grade I) 92 (T1 Grade I)	—	[95]

[a] TIS only = 83%

S, single; M, multiple

invasive bladder tumors. Although series differ, the incidence of subsequent development of invasive tumors in superficial bladder cancer patients is in the range of 7%–10% [55, 91, 96, 138, 143, 188]. The results of studies evaluating tumor recurrence, invasion, and survival are summarized in Table 2. The avoidance of this invasive event is the purpose of all treatments, surgical or chemotherapeutic, in the management of superficial bladder cancer.

Grade

The histologic grade of the tumor has been demonstrated to have an impact on the 5-year survival rates in patients with superficial bladder cancers, even when stage is considered. The grade of bladder neoplasm provides the clinician with an estimate of the potential for growth and subsequent invasion of the bladder wall, the probabilty of which increases with increasing tumor grade. It was long ago that Broders described the initial grading concept for bladder carcinomas. He recognized four tumor grades, placing the least aggressive papillomas (grade I) at one end of the spectrum, increasing to the most malignant grades (grade IV) at the other end [15]. It has become common practice to refer to grades I and II as low-grade tumors and grades III and IV as high-grade tumors. As tumor grade increases, survival appears to diminish. Barnes and associates [9] found that the grade of tumor was an important factor affecting survival. In their series, the reported 5-year survival rate was 85% for those patients with grade I tumors in contrast to a 51% survival rate for those with grade II tumors. The 5-year survival rate of the grade I neoplasm patients did not differ significantly from the general population (85% versus 87%, $p > 0.05$). Nichols and Marshall [122] also found a difference in survival rate which correlated to tumor grade. The survival rate for low-grade tumors was better than for high-grade tumors (82.6% versus 76.6%) at 5-year follow-up. Grade may however be a less important determinant of recurrence when compared to stage. Lutzeyer et al. [95, 150] in a series of 315 patients found recurrence rates of 52%, 69%, and 77% in patients with stages Ta, T1, T2, respectively, whereas the recurrence rates by grade were 63%, 67%, and 71% for grades I, II, III tumors, respectively. However, an observation by this group was that grade was an influencing factor in recurrences occurring at a higher grade or stage. Of those with grades I, II, and III tumors, 20%, 37%, and 64%, respectively, recurred at a higher grade or stage.

Multicentricity

There is a great deal of controversy in the literature as to whether those patients with single versus multiple lesions have a different prognosis. Lerman et al. [91] found a recurrence rate of 31% in patients with single papillomas against 66% in those with multiple lesions. These results are in accordance with other investigators [104, 170]. The progression to bladder cancer was significantly greater in patients with multiple papillomas (13.6% versus 4.6%). Greene and associates [55] reviewed grade I tumors and reported a high recurrence rate in both single and multiple tumor presentations (68% and 88%, respectively), where Williams and co-workers [188] studied T1 bladder tumors in 167 patients and found a higher incidence of subsequent invasion into the lamina propria in patients with multiple tumors (44%) versus single tumors

(21%). The overall survival rate was 72%, with little difference noted between patients with single or multiple tumors. More recently, Lutzeyer and associates [95] analyzed a series of 315 patients. During a 3-year follow-up period, the overall recurrence rate was 64%. The recurrence rate for solitary tumors was 46%, while that for multiple tumors was 73%. Tumor progression was studied in 274 cases. The progression rate was highest in patients with multiple tumors of both the Ta and T1 types with progression rates of 43% and 46%, respectively. To date, the results reported from the larger series suggest that those patients with multiple tumors have a higher recurrence rate and a higher incidence of subsequent bladder wall invasion, but the impact of these findings on survival is not well documented.

Carcinoma in situ

Another important factor in the natural and therapeutic history of superficial bladder cancer is the presence of carcinoma in situ. Carcinoma in situ is a different biologic entity in that it probably represents a spectrum of neoplasia. There are at least four different clinical situations which may have very different biologic outcomes: 1) a small foci of carcinoma in situ immediately adjacent to a papilloma of the bladder; 2) a number of areas on random biopsy which show carcinoma in situ at the time of TUR of a papilloma; 3) total or near total involvement of the urothelium with carcinoma in situ, with or without papillary tumors; 4) symptomatic (irritative bladder symptoms) carcinoma in situ, which is associated with total or near total mucosal involvement. Melicow in 1952 [103] reported the presence of epithelial hyperplasia, squamous metaplasia, and carcinoma in situ in perfectly normal regions of bladders removed from ten patients; it was some 8−10 years later that the potentially serious nature of this incidental finding of carcinoma in situ became evident. At least 80% of bladders removed surgically for invasive disease show carcinoma in situ or multifocal carcinoma [28, 48, 87, 104, 117, 147, 165]. Eisenberg and associates [44] revealed a 26% incidence of carcinoma in situ in areas adjacent to papillary tumors. Later, Schade and Swinney [153] detected a 40% incidence of carcinoma in situ in similar biopsies. Wallace's group [184] found a variable frequency of carcinoma in biopsies of apparently normal urothelium. This seemingly normal mucosa revealed a 33% incidence of histologic abnormalities including 4.5% with carcinoma (papillary or invasive). Red, flat mucosa showing a 52% incidence of histologic abnormality included 14% with carcinoma, while granular or mossy like mucosa revealed a 42% incidence of carcinoma. In a more recent survey, Soloway et al. [162] found a 46% incidence of atypia, 16% incidence of carcinoma, and 14% rate of carcinoma in situ from these cystoscopically normal looking areas of the bladder. Althausen and associates [3] found that later development of infiltrating cancer correlated with the morphology of the mucous membrane immediately adjacent to the papillary tumor. The incidence of invasive bladder carcinoma in less than 5 years was 7% in patients with normal adjacent urothelium, 36% in patients with atypical mucous membrane, and 83% in patients with carcinoma in situ adjacent to the papilloma. These findings suggest that some of these proliferative areas may progress to neoplasia, and there appears to be a somewhat worse prognosis for the patient population with focal proliferative areas of involvement versus those with no such involvement during initial TUR of papillary tumor of the bladder. These findings have led to the conclusion that the evaluation of the entire bladder urothelium should be performed through the utilization of multiple mucosal biopsies at the time of initial primary tumor resection [184]. Carcinoma in situ may also extend beyond the bladder into the prostatic urethra and prostatic ducts [49, 154, 158]. Autopsy evidence of in situ urethral cancer has been found in 18%–19% of patients who died of bladder cancer [54, 174]. The risk of developing upper tract tumors is present in about 5% of cases, and the development of urethral tumors occurs in about 5%–10% of patients [49, 54, 154, 158]. Recognition and control of these tumors by nonsurgical means is difficult. The recognition of particularly the latter of the above-mentioned clinical situations as being distinct in its biologic behavior is recent. Symptomatic diffuse carcinoma in situ of the bladder has been associated with a 50%–80% incidence of infiltrating cancer [48, 49, 173]. This clinical entity represents a dangerous extreme in the spectrum of disease observed with carcinoma in situ, and cystectomy may generally be indicated following the assessment of multicentricity, grade of tumor, and location of tumor growth.

Tumor Implantation

The concept of tumor implantation is another factor that may influence the natural of therapeutic history of superficial bladder cancer. Although this phenomenon is difficult, if not impossible, to prove, laboratory animal studies and circumstantial evidence in humans provide evidence that this factor may exist. Tumor implantation has been demonstrated in dogs by McDonald and Thorsen [102], by Wallace and Herschfiels using a rat sarcoma model [182], and through a syngeneic murine model by Weldon and Soloway [185]. Facors discussed previously such as multicentricity, tumor grade, stage, presence of carcinoma in situ, or other determinants such as incomplete excision of the primary tumor, understaging, occult prostatic or urethral involvement, or continued exposure to carcinogens, all influence and limit any conclusions which may be made concerning tumor implantation in the human bladder. Urethral or bladder neck recurrences led a number of investigators to consider implantation as an etiologic factor in new occurrences of bladder tumors [52, 59, 62, 82]. Hollands [65] reported a 3% incidence of urethral tumors when studying recurrent tumors versus a 0.3% incidence in initial tumors. It was also noted that the wound recurrence rate was higher following segmental resection as against transvesical fulguration (10% of 224 transvesical fulgurations versus 19.5% of 118 segmental resections). Hollands thus emphasized tumor cell implantation in both the urethra and traumatized urothelium as a factor in recurrence rates. Other circumstantial evidence supporting tumor implantation as an etiologic factor in tumor recurrence is provided by Burnand et al. [18]. These investigators found a significant decrease in the recurrence rate after 1 year between a treatment group receiving 90 mg thiotepa intravesically for 30 min following TUR versus a nonchemotherapy control group (58% versus 97% recurrence, respectively). It is unlikely that a single intravesical dose of thiotepa would alter the development of new tumors, and the decrease in recurrence rate in the treatment group was felt to be due to prevention of a viable tumor implanting into the urothelium. Veenema and associates [180] also instilled thiotepa into the wound and bladder at the time of surgery. No tumor implantation into the wound was noted during an average follow-up time of 2 years. Similar evidence has been reported by van der Werf-Messing [177]. This study utilized radium implants to control large superficial tumors, which are unlikely to eradicate tumor at distant sites. The reported recurrence rates with radium-treated patients was 12% in contrast to the 50%

recurrence rate in those patients treated by TUR alone. It was thought that the local therapy with radium prevented tumor implantation in the local therapy with radium prevented tumor implantation in the traumatized bladder mucosa. Although strong evidence for support of the phenomenon of tumor implantation may be impossible to provide due to the multiplicity of factors influencing tumor recurrence, this concept should be considered a possibility in light of the current circumstantial evidence.

The Endoscopic Evaluation Procedure

Bladder tumors are rarely found as incidental findings in an asymptomatic patient in a routine physical examination or at autopsy. Most frequently, hematuria and irritative bladder symptoms predominate at the initial presentation. In patients with carcinoma in situ, it has been reported that 90% of patients will have symptoms of frequency, dysuria, urgency, and hematuria [174]. Treatment of superficial bladder cancer is dependent upon a complete evaluation of the grade and extent of the tumor. The therapeutic decision is influenced by findings on excretory urogram, urinary cytology, and transurethral examination. The initial endoscopic (transurethral) examination includes the visualization of the bladder mucosa. If the bladder tumor is visualized, resection and/or fulguration is made, with an attempt made to leave a free margin at the base of the tumor. Random biopsies of the bladder mucosa have been suggested at this time [184], as well as bimanual examination under anesthesia. Patients are routinely cystoscoped every 3 months following the initial examination to evaluate the possibility of recurrent tumors in the bladder. Should patients become symptomatic at a time earlier than the 3-monthly interval, they should be recystoscoped. Although subsequent cystoscopies are not usually carried out under general anesthesia, there is a low but significant morbidity in this costly and invasive procedure. The efficacy of the use of recurrent symptomology, such as visible hematuria or irritable bladder symptoms, or of recurrent laboratory abnormalities, such as microscopic hematuria or bladder cytology as a threshold for recystoscopic examination has never been examined. The timing in relation to the patient's benefit of the repeat urologic procedures has never been formally addressed to our knowledge.

Rationale for Intravesical Bladder Chemotherapy

Since recurrence of superficial tumors is frequent, even with complete surgical resection, adjuvant therapies have been utilized for some time. Intravesical (topical) chemotherapy is an attractive mode of therapy for a variety of reasons: 1) an antineoplastic agent instilled into the bladder would allow a high concentration of the drug to come into contact with the urothelium for a relatively long period of time; 2) this route might also allow a reduced likelihood of tumor recurrence by destroying viable tumor cells in the bladder following TUR and thus prevent tumor implantation; 3) it might also exert cytotoxic activity on residual carcinoma or on carcinoma in situ adjacent to a papilloma; 4) it might minimize systemic toxicity to the agent; 5) it might delay or abort the need for cystectomy and attendant loss of urinary and sexual function in what may be an asymptomatic patient.

Background and History

Intravesical chemotherapy of superficial bladder tumors appears to be as old as medical cancer therapy. The first report of this type of therapy began with Herring's report on the use of silver nitrate in 1903 [60]. Since this citation, some 23 agents have been employed to treat superficial bladder tumors (Table 3). Compounds such as silver nitrate [60], trichloroacetic acid [79], podophyllin [39, 157], and oxochlorosene [151] are no longer used.

Radioactive solution such as gold-198 [35], arsenic-76 [43], sodium [183], bromine [183], and yttrium-90 [40] have displayed little activity. Of the 'modern day' cancer chemotherapeutic agents that have been investigated in intravesical chemotherapy, those agents no longer used because of toxicity or lack of therapeutic effect include actinomycin-D [47], 5-fluorouracil [47], methotrexate [1], cyclophosphamide [135], nitrogen mustard [135], and bleomycin [14, 160]. Recently, Needles and associates have reported the lack of effect of cisplatin in controlling recurrent TIS and T1 bladder cancer [121]. Recent studies have provided evidence for the potential usefulness of a number of chemotherapeutic agents via the intravesical route. These agents include thiotepa, epodyl, mitomycin-C, doxorubicin, bacillus Calmette-Guerin, and teniposide (VM-26). The remainder of the discussion will focus on the utility of these agents in the treatment and prophylaxis of superficial bladder cancer.

Table 3. Agents previously used for intravesical therapy of bladder cancer

Agent	Year	Author	Reference no.
Silver nitrate	1903	Herring	[60]
Trichloroacetic acid	1919	Joseph	[79]
Podophyllin	1948	Semple	[157]
	1950	Duckworth	[39]
Gold-198	1960	Dickson	[35]
Thiotepa	1961	Jones	[78]
Oxochlorosene	1963	Russell	[151]
Arsenic-76	1964	Einhorn	[43]
Actinomycin-D	1965	Esquival	[47]
5-Fluorouracil	1965	Esquival	[47]
Methotrexate	1966	Abassian	[1]
Mannitol myleran	1966	Abassian	[1]
Cyclophosphamide	1970	Pavone-Macaluso	[135]
Nitrogen mustard	1970	Pavone-Macaluso	[135]
Peptochemio	1970	Pavone-Macaluso	[135]
Radioactive sodium	1971	Wallace	[183]
Radioactive bromine	1971	Wallace	[183]
Epodyl	1971	Riddle	[145]
Doxorubicin	1972	Pavone-Macaluso	[133]
Bleomycin	1973	Sadoughi	[152]
Yttrium-90	1975	Durrant	[40]
Mitomycin-C	1975	Mishina	[108]
Bacillus Calmette-Guerin	1976	Morales	[111]
Teniposide (VM-26)	1978	Pavone-Macaluso	[135]

Pharmacologic Considerations

As stated earlier, the rational for intravesical bladder chemotherapy is to provide antineoplastic agents to the tumor at a higher concentration than achievable by systemic administration of the drug and to do so with minimal systemic absorption, and hence, systemic toxicity to the patient. Although the bladder is permeable to a variety of substances such as urea, water, sodium, and chloride ions [97], this is seldom thought to be of clinical significance. The impermeability of the bladder urothelium is thought to be based on the ultrastructural findings of the asymmetric membrane linked by desmasomes on the luminal side of the urothelial surface cell [161], the tight junctions connecting the umbrella cells, and the basement membrane [11, 86, 105]. The five major factors that influence the absorption of drug through the three cellular layers of the bladder as well as the three elements listed above are molecular weight of the drug, alterations in the urothelial surface, pH of the solution, which controls the polarity of the agent, drug concentration, and time of drug exposure to the urothelial surface.

The molecular weight of the compound appears to be an important factor in allowing absorption of an agent into the bloodstream. Maluf [97] found that the bladder acted as a poorly permeable membrane, allowing absorption of some chemicals such as urea, water, sodium, and chloride ions. The absorptive process was that of passive diffusion. Work with various sulfonamides has indicated that the molecular weigth is a significant factor in allowing absorption of the urothelium by this class of compounds. It appeared that substances with molecular weights greater than 200 were not absorbed to any appreciable amount, while those compounds with molecular weights (MW) less than 200 were absorbed by passive diffusion [78]. However, molecular weight is not the sole factor to be considered in evaluating the absorbability of a compound, as leukopenia has been a systemic toxicity noted following the instillation of methotrexate (an antineoplastic agent with MW of 454.5) into the bladder.

Alteration in the urothelium is another significant factor influencing the ability of an agent to gain access to the vascular bed. As cancerous changes progress, it has been demonstrated that the asymmetric unit membrane progressively loses its differentiation. Increases in thiotepa absorption rates apparently occur early when dedifferentiation may only be noted by electron microscopy [61]. Transurethral resection has been shown to dramatically increases the absorption of thiotepa and doxorubicin when these agents are instilled into the bladder within 1 week of resection. Mean absorptions were 73% for thiotepa and 62% for doxorubicin [134]. The presence of bladder mucosa inflammation also acts to increase drug absorption, such as that following instrumentation, diathermy, or infection.

The effect of the pH on the absorption of chemotherapeutic agents in the bladder has not been well studied. Pharmacologically, it is well known that when the pH of a solution exceeds the pKa of the agent, the nonionized (absorbable) species of the drug predominates. For doxorubicin, Eksborg et al. [45] recommended the use of a phosphate buffer as a vehicle for administration of the agent into the bladder to prevent the large fluctuations in pH observed during instillation with saline. The pKa of doxorubicin is 8.2; at pHs above 8.2, the nonionized form predominates, potentially facilitating absorption of the drug, and at higher pHs, the drug may undergo degradation. The concept of using suitable buffers is novel and should be evaluated in future investigations. Since smaller molecular weight drugs are absorbed through the bladder by passive diffusion, the concentration gradient of the agent between the plasma and the solution contained in the bladder is a critical factor in the absorptive process. Some investigators have suggested that threatment for each patient be based on concentration, rather than dose. Eksborg and associates [45] have suggested measuring bladder capacity and instilling a volume of drug into the bladder equal to the bladder capacity minus 50 ml. Thus the concentration would remain constant for each patient but the dose and total volume per instillation would vary. However, it must be noted that patients may find it impossible to retain this large quantity of a drug solution volume for the prescribed amount of time (1–2 h).

The time that the drug is in contact with the urothelium may also influence the amount of drug that may penetrate the bladder and enter the systemic circulation. A good deal of evaluation is needed in this area. The optimal contact time has not been studied in any controlled fashion, neither have the frequency of instillations or the utility of other methods of administration, such as continuous irrigations [27]. The influence that ancillary agents, such as urokinase [64], increased viscosity solutions, or dimethyl-sulfoxide, exert on tumor penetration, bladder penetration, efficacy, or toxicity is unknown. Other areas of uncertainty include the utility of multiple drug regimens or sequential use of agents to gain cell synchronization, the role of biologic response modifiers alone or in combination with chemotherapeutic agents, and the use of chemoprotectants such as retinoic acid. Some of these concepts may become less significant in light of recent data indicating that the histologic changes associated with the intravesical use of chemotherapeutic agents may not be cytotoxic and inhibition DNA replication, but rather acting as substances toxic to the urothelium, causing increased exfoliation with denudation of the papillary and/or flat urothelium [116].

Absorption studies of the most commonly used chemotherapeutic agents for instillation into the bladder are reviewed in Table 4. Jones and Swinney [78] found that 33% of a dose of thiotepa (MW = 189) was absorbed following a 30 mg intravesical dose which was retained for 3 h. This is consistent with the frequent leukopenia that has been observed in the clinical studies performed thus far. Studies evaluating the absorption of doxorubicin (MW = 580) have produced discordant results. Jacobi and Kurth [70] found trace amounts of doxorubicin in the serum of seven patients, five of which were tumor free, and two of which had tumor recurrence. Lundbeck and associates [94] found that most patients absorbed 4% of an intravesical dose. Pavone-Macaluso [134] has reported up to 93.7% drug absorption if the doxorubicin was administered within 1 week of TUR. During routine bladder instillations, absorption rates were found to be 17%–58% for a 30-mg dose and 20%–67% for a 60-mg dose. Most investigators have not observed any systemic toxicity symptoms during intravesical therapy with doxorubicin [70, 94]. Mitomycin-C (MW = 334) appears to afford little systemic absorption, and hence toxicity, as both Mishina and associates [109] and De Furia et al. [32] found that only trace amounts of the drug were absorbed into the systemic circulation following doses of 20–60 mg (the time between surgical procedure and drug instillation was not stated). Neither investigator found any clinical toxicity. In considering the risk of systemic toxicity from the instillation of chemotherapeutic agents into the bladder, doxorubicin and mitomycin-C are absorbed into the systemic circulation to a much lesser degree than thiotepa and are less toxic alternatives. One must keep in mind the factors discussed above which influence toxicity, such as TUR, that may drastically alter the absorption capability of an agent when instilled into the bladder. In drug selection the sensitivity of the tumor of the chemotherapeutic agent should be kept in mind if such information is available [31].

Table 4. Systemic absorption of chemotherapeutic agents from the bladder

Author	Drug	Dose	Retention time (h)	Range % absorption	AVG % absorption
Jones [78]	Thiotepa	30 mg/ 100 ml	3	33	33
Pavone-Macaluso [134]	Doxorubicin	30 mg	2	17–58	–
		60 mg	2	20–67	–
Pavone-Macaluso [134]	Doxorubicin	Post-TUR	2	39–94	62
Lundbeck [94]	Doxorubicin	100 mg/ 100 ml	1	0–16	4
Jacobi [70]	Doxorubicin	40 mg/ 30 ml	2	Trace	Trace
Mishina [109]	Mitomycin	20 mg/ 20 ml	1	Trace	Trace
De Furia [32]	Mitomycin	20–60 mg	2	None	None
Leissner [90]	5-FU	250 mg	3	None	None

Thiotepa

Thiotepa is a polyfunctional alkylating agent chemically related to nitrogen mustard. Following formation of ethylenimine radicals, alkylation of purine and pyrimidine bases with crosslinking between DNA, DNA and RNA, nucleic acids, and proteins occurs. The net effect is inhibition of DNA, RNA, and nucleic acid synthesis. Thiotepa is not cell-cycle specific.

Numerous reports [1, 18, 19, 38, 41, 47, 67, 84, 110, 123, 127, 130, 132, 181, 186] have evaluated the usefulness of thiotepa instillations in superficial bladder following the initial report of Jones and Swinney [78], which demonstrated the ability of the agent to destroy superficial bladder tumors with little or no adverse effect on the normal urothelium. When used as definite therapy for low-grade superficial bladder tumors, approximately one-third of patients will respond completely, one-third will show partial regressions, and one-third will show no respone (Table 5). Although it is generally agreed that prophylactic doses should be employed following initial definite therapy, there has not been an extensive amount of long term follow-up data until recently. Esquivel et al. [47] observed that all three of their patients had recurrences within 6–7 months following complete disappearance of papilloma after 4–12 weekly thiotepa instillations when therapy was discontinued. Oristavo [130] found recurrences in 50% of patients within 6 months if intravesical therapy was not continued in his patients. These early studies provided the stimulus to study the effectiveness of prophylactic thiotepa instilled into the bladder following definitive therapy with either TUR or thiotepa. A number of the larger series performed to date have demonstrated the ability of prophylactic therapy to reduce the recurrence rate and/or increase the time up to recurrence following definitive therapy with TUR, fulguration, or intravesical therapy (Table 6). Koontz and associates [84] reported the finding of the National Bladder Cancer Collaborative Group. The prophylaxis study encompassed 93 patients, which compromised a quite heterogeneous group as far as history, number of previous, invasion into the lamina propria, and existence of multifocal tumors. The doses of thiotepa employed were 30 and 60 mg instilled into the bladder no earlier than 3 weeks following resection of a superficial tumor. The frequency of administration was every 4 weeks. After 12 months and 20 months, the percentage of patients free of tumors was significantly greater for the treatment group than the control group (66% against 40% at 12 months, and 54% against 28% at 20 months, respectively). Results for the 30-mg dose were similar to those for the 60-mg dose. Of note was that patients who were successfully treated for incompletely resected tumors with thiotepa, 100% were disease-free after 12 months.

Soloway [163] reviewed the results of the EORTC Genitourinary Tract Cancer Cooperative Group [156]; 215 patients with T1 tumors were randomized to thiotepa, VM-26, or to no treatment following TUR. Therapy was started 4 weeks after resection and administered weekly for 4 weeks and then monthly. There was no difference between treatment groups in the time of first recurrence; however, thiotepa was able to reduce significantly the recurrence rate as compared to VM-26 or controls.

Another means of providing prophylactic activity is to instill thiotepa into the bladder at the time of the operative procedure. The rationale for this therapy is to prevent recurrence as a consequence of tumor-cell implantation into the wound or bladder wall. Veenema and associates [181] instilled thiotepa solutions into the bladder at the time of operation in 20 patients. Over a 2-year average follow-up period, no tumor implants into the wound occurred. Burnand et al. [18] found that a 30-min, 90-mg instillation of thiotepa into the bladder immediately post-TUR lowered the incidence of recurrent bladder tumors. Patients were followed-up for a period of 2−5 years. Eight of 19 patients remained free of tumor recurrence ($p < 0.001$). Only one of the treatment patients became leukopenic. Gavrell and his group [53] also studied the effect of thiotepa postsurgically. Each patient served as his/her own control. Two treatment groups were formed from the study population. The first group received 30 mg thiotepa for 30 min twice daily for 3 days starting on the day of surgery. The other treatment group received the same initial therapy as the first group but also received an additional weekly dose for 6 weeks, then at monthly intervals for 1 year, and then every 3 months thereafter. Prior to therapy, the patients averaged one recurrence every 9.5 months. The first treatment group averaged one recurrence every 33 months, while the second treatment group averaged one recurrence per 41 months. Only 2 of 22 patients became leukopenic. This mode of prophylaxis appears to be a safe and effective mode of therapy for tumor implantation as long as the bladder urothelium is not excessively traumatized by extensive resection and/or fulguration.

Overall, the prophylactic studies outlined in Table 5 appear to decrease the incidence of patients with recurrence and/or decrease the frequency of recurrences as compared to a control population. Failures in prophylactic therapy with intravesical thiotepa probably have an early recurrence. Nieh and associates [123] studied a prophylaxis regimen in 93 patients. Of 16 failures (nine control, seven treatment), 11 were detected at the first follow-up cystoscopy at 3 months. A later report by the same group [127] found that in eight patients who had residual tumor post-TUR eradicated by intravesical thiotepa and were subsequently placed on prophylactic therapy, tumor recurrence occurred after 6−27 months (average 15.1 months). In contrast, the untreated group showed recurrence after 2−9 months (average 4.3 months).

Thiotepa is usually administered at a dose of 30−60 mg at a 1-mg/ml concentration. The schedule of administration is highly variable. In definitive therapy, schedules have

Table 5. Thiopeta response as definitive therapy of superficial bladder cancer

Author	Patients no.	Complete response no. (%)	Partial response no. (%)	No response no. (%)
Jones 1961 [78]	13	0 (0)	11 (85)	2 (15)
Esquivel 1965 [47]	10	3 (30)	4 (40)	3 (30)
Abbassian 1966 [1]	13	3 (23)	5 (38)	5 (38)
Veenema 1969 [181]	46	17 (37)	16 (35)	13 (28)
Edsmyr 1970 [41]	29	12 (41)	12 (41)	5 (17)
Pavone-Macaluso 1971 [132]	25	8 (32)	8 (32)	9 (36)
Koontz 1981 [84]	95	45 (47)	–	50 (53)
	231	88 (38)	56 (24)	87 (38)

ranged from a dose four times per week over a 1-week period [84] to weekly doses [47, 181] followed by monthly doses. In prophylactic therapy, the most common schedule is a weekly dose given four times, followed by a monthly dose thereafter [19, 41, 186]. The drug should be administered into an empty bladder via a catheter. It is expedient that the patient restrict fluid intake for a period of 8–12 h prior to therapy to minimize diuresis-dilution of the drug in the bladder and to aid in the ability of the patient to retain the drug in the bladder for the advocated 2-h contact time. The patient should also rotate his position every 15 min to insure that the entire bladder urothelium comes in contact with the drug solution. Recommended patient care procedures are listed in Table 12.

Because the mw of thiotepa is low (189), the drug is absorbed into the systemic circulation. Alteration of the integrity of the bladder urothelium by factors discussed earlier also plays an important role in the passage of the drug through the urothelium into the systemic circulation. Absorption of thiotepa was found by Jones and Swinney [78] to be 33% of an administered dose, whereas Pavone-Macaluso found it to be up to 73% of a dose if thiotepa was instilled into bladder within 1 week of TUR. In any case, it becomes clinically apparent that the absorption of thiotepa is a significant factor in modulating toxicity. The major toxicity of thiotepa is bone marrow suppression, which may be manifest as leukopenia or thrombocytopenia. The incidence of this toxicity ranges from 2%–26% [65, 66, 78] and, at times, may be fatal [1, 41]. Bladder contracture and chemical cystitis may also be noted. Urinary tract infection with symptoms of irritation or dysuria has been noted in 2%–40% of patients. This is probably a manifestation of frequent catheterization, and palliation through the use of prophylactic antimicrobial agents may be indicated. In one study, an incidence of 3% allergic drug reactions (5 of 164 patients) was observed with manifestations of fever, hives, pruritis, or angioneurotic edema [181]. All of these patients had a past medical history of allergies to other drugs.

Thiotepa is commercially available in the United States from Lederle Laboratories as 15-mg vials. Intact vials should be stored under refrigeration (2°–8° C). Each vial, when reconstitued with 15 ml sterile water yields a 1-mg/ml solution. The reconstituted solution is stable chemically for a period of 5 days. However, as no preservatives are added, the unused portion should be discarded in 24 h. Solutions should be clear; any opaque solutions should not be used [36]. The average wholesale price of thiotepa is $ 8.10 for a 15-mg vial, $ 16.20 for a 30-mg dose, and $ 32.40 for a 60-mg dose [6].

Table 6. Results of thiopeta prophylaxis

Author	Patients no.	% Recurrence		Follow-up time	Average time to recurrence treatment
		Control	Treatment		
Westcott 1966 [186]	14	75	0	Variable	
Pavone-Macaluso 1971 [132]	14	60	21	1 year (mean)	
Drew 1968 [38]	6	–	33	18 months +	130 weeks
Burnand 1976 [18]	51	97	58	2–5 years	2.2 months
Byar 1977 [19]	121	60	47	$\bar{x}$.31 months	
Koontz 1981 [84]	93	60	40	2 years	
Schulman [156]	224	52	49	NS	

NS, not stated

Ethoglucid (Epodyl)

Ethoglucid (Epodyl, triethyleneglycol diglycidyl ether) is a diepoxide alkylating agent widely used in Europe. The mw of this agent is 262.3 as compared to a mw of thiotepa of 189. This difference in mw is thought to be the explanation for the clinical observation of less systemic side effects of the former drug. Clinical trials in Europe [1, 26, 50, 124, 144, 146, 148, 159] indicate that ethoglucid is an active drug in the treatment of superficial bladder tumors. Overall, it appears that the activity of this agent is equivalent, if not slightly superior, to that of thiotepa (Table 7). However, these two agents have never been compared in any randomized fashion. Approximately 45% of patients will acheive a complete response and 25% a partial response, producing an overall response rate of 70%. The length of follow-up times and the numbers of patients discontinuing treatment because of cystitis are important factors to be considered when evaluating the effectiveness of ethoglucid. Riddle and Wallace [146] found, during a 3-year follow-up period, a trend indicating that the majority of patients who achieve a complete response tend to maintain it. The increases in nonresponders over a period of time generally involves leaving the partial response category. A similar trend was also noted by Smith et al. [159]. Koontz and associates [84] also noted a similar trend with thiotepa. The number of patients who discontinue ethoglucid intravesical therapy because of chemical cystitis becomes an important factor in the statistical analysis of the effectiveness of this agent. Nielsen and Thybo [124] found that 16% of the 44 patients in their study group had discontinued therapy because of cystitis. If the patients with cystitis remain in the statistical analysis (as nonresponders), the overall response rate (complete response + partial response, CR + PR) is 43%; if only those patients able to complete the course of therapy are evaluated, the overall response rate would be 53%. A similar problem was also noted by Colleen and associates [26] who lost 10 of 39 patients for further treatment due to cystitis.

Ethoglucid is usually administered as a 1% solution by instillation into the bladder through a urethral catheter with a 1-h retention time. The most commonly used schedules have been to start with 12 doses of a weekly schedule, followed by monthly

Table 7. Epodyl response in superficial bladder cancer

Author	Patients no.	Complete response no. (%)	Partial response no. (%)	No response no. (%)	Follow-up time (months)
Abassian 1966 [1]	15	5 (33)	3 (20)	7 (47)	NS[a]
Riddle 1973 [146]	64	38 (59)	24 (38)	2 (3)	3
Robinson 1977 [148]	41	17 (41)	18 (44)	6 (15)	3
Smith 1978 [159]	12	8 (67)	3 (25)	1 (8)	6
Fitzpatrick 1979 [50]	64	19 (30)	20 (32)	24 (38)	12
Nielsen 1979 [124]	44	16 (36)	3 (7)	25 (57)[b]	3
Colleen 1980 [26]	39	23 (58)	NS[a]	16 (42)	6
	279	126 (45)	71 (25)	81 (29)	5.5 (AVG)

[a] Not stated
[b] Includes patients discontinued because of cystitis

doses for 1 year, then progressing to a schedule of every 3 months thereafter if a response is noted.

Although actual absorption rates of ethoglucid in the bladder have not been determined, clinical studies indicate that it undergoes significantly less systemic absorption than thiotepa. Severe leukopenia is rareley observed [148]. Moderate irritative symptoms may be observed in about one-half of patients [1], urinary frequency and urgency in 25%−50% [1, 148], which may lead to discontinuation of therapy in less than 10% of patients [50, 159], and chemical cystitis of such severity so as to preclude further therapy in 16%−25% of patients [26, 124]. Other observed side effects have included painful urination in about one-third [148], bladder contracture in 20%, and rarely, an allergic reaction [50].

Ethoglucid is not commercially available in the United States. It is available in Europe as Epodyl (ICI Pharmaceuticals) in 1-ml vials. Solutions for instillation into the bladder should be made fresh, as the drug may lose potency and react with plastics at high concentrations [100]. The drug may be diluted in sterile water for irrigation.

Mitomycin-C

Mitomycin-C (Mutamycin, Bristol Laboratories) is a purple-colored antibiotic derived from *Streptomyces caespitosus*. This agent is activated intracellularly through enzymatic reduction of the quinone group and loss of a methoxy group, which results in the production of a bifunctional or trifunctional alkylating agent. These active metabolites are then able to crosslink DNA, degrade performed DNA, and inhibit DNA synthesis [36].

A number of trials have been performed with mitomycin-C following the initial results of Mishina and associates [108] in Japan (Table 8). Their observations in 50 patients were a 44% complete response rate and a 32% partial response rate, producing an overall response of 76%. The lack of bone marrow toxicity was of interest. The largest series to date in the United States, reported by De Furia et al. [32], supported

Table 8. Mitomycin-C response in superficial bladder cancer

Author	Patients no.	Complete response no. (%)	Partial response no. (%)	No response no. (%)
Mishina 1975 [108]	33[a]	20 (61)	9 (27)	4 (12)
Kaufmann 1979 [80]	8	5 (63)	3 (37)	0 (0)
De Furia 1980 [32][b]	55	25 (45)	12 (22)	18 (33)
Camuzzi 1980 [20][b]	32	32 (100)	0 (0)	4 (12)
Prout 1981 [142][b]	22	13 (59)	–	9 (52)
Issel 1981 [68][c]	37	13 (35)	9 (24)	15 (41)
	187	108 (58)	33 (18)	46 (24)

[a] Data excludes patients in study with stage B1-D disease
[b] Data includes thiopeta failures
[c] All patients = thiopeta failures

Mishina's earlier findings. An overall response rate of 67% was noted, with a 45% complete response rate and a 22% partial response rate. Of interest was that eight of nine patients (89%) who failed prior to intravesical chemotherapy, eight had complete responses. The doses ranged from 20–60 mg, and no clear-cut dose-response was noted, although not all groups were evaluable due to insufficient follow-up time. The authors concluded that the duration of complete response (CR) was longer than that observed for thiotepa. However, mitomycin-C in this series had a median duration CR of 14.5 months, which is comparable to the findings with thiotepa by Nocks et al. [127], who found that 8 of 18 patients who showed recurrence total ablation of residual tumor with thiotepa and subsequent prophylactic therapy, did so in an average of 15.1 months. These results need verification in a prospective randomized trial in a larger population size. Mitomycin-C does appear to have significant activity in thiotepa failures. In addition to the eight of nine patients reported above who responded to mitomycin-C following prior intravesical therapy, Camuzzi and associates [20] found they were able to control 100% of superficial bladder tumors in 32 patients, of which 21 were thiotepa failures. The mean follow-up time was 18 months. Prout et al. [142] observed six CRs in a group of 13 thiotepa failures. These patients remained tumor-free for an average of 9 months. The CR in de novo patients of in patients with previous successful thiotepa therapy was 89% (eight of nine patients). Issel's group [68] studied mitomycin-C activity in 37 thiotepa refractory patients. Of these, 35% achieved CR and 25% a partial response. Similar to the findings of significant recurrence following termination of thiotepa therapy [47, 130], mitomycin-C appears also to require maintenance therapy. Soloway and associates [164] found that following an initial CR to definitive mitomycin-C therapy, eight patients remained in CR if they completed a 1-year maintenance program of monthly mitomycin-C; however, after discontinuing the program, five (64%) developed superficial tumor in 6–8 months. The response rates for mitomycin-C appear to be of the order of about a 76% overall response rate with approximately 60% of patients achieving a CR rate and 20% a partial response rate.

Because of the negligible absorption of mitomycin-C from the bladder, little systemic toxicity is evident in the clinical studies performed thus far (Table 4). There have been no reported cases of systemic toxicity (bone marrow depression) with the instillation of mitomycin-C into the bladder. Local effects of mitomycin-C also seem to be mild. The most common side effect is bladder irritation, which occurs in about 10%−15% of patients [68, 126, 142] and may require termination of therapy [142]. Palmar rash of the hands may occur in 5%−15% of patients [32, 68, 126] and may be resolved with oral antihistamines and topical corticosteroids, as it appears to be a contact dermatitis. Washing the hands and perineum can prevent this occurrence. One patient developed a generalized rash with palmar rash [126]. Dysuria and frequency may respond to temporary discontinuation of the drug or with appropriate treatment of infection [126].

The doses of mitomycin-C utilized have ranged from 20−60 mg, usually administered as a 1-mg/ml concentration in sterile water. The schedule most commonly encountered is a weekly interval with eight instillations. The administration technique is similar to that for thiotepa. The desired dose is administered through a urethral catheter, and the contents are held in the bladder for a 2-h period. Mitomycin-C is available in 5-mg and 20-mg vials (Mutamycin, Bristol Laboratories). The drug may be stored at room temperature prior to use. For bladder instillation, the drug may be reconstituted in sterile water. It should be protected from light if not used within 24 h. The drug is stable for 14 days when refrigerated and for 7 days at room temperature [36]. The cost of the drug (at direct cost from the manufacturer) Is $ 35.44 per 5-mg vial and $ 131.68 per 20-mg vial. This equates to about $ 132 for a 20-mg dose, $ 264 for a 40-mg dose, and $ 396 for a 60-mg dose [6]. This is a significant cost difference when compared to thiotepa or doxorubicin.

Doxorubicin (Adriamycin)

Doxorubicin is an anthracycline antibiotic antineoplastic agent obtained from the bacterium *Streptomyces peucetius var. caesius.* It is a hydroxylated form of daunorubicin. Structurally, it contains a water-soluble basic-reducing sugar daunosamine, linked via a glycosidic bond to the water-insoluble tetracyclic compound adriamycinone. The anthracycline class of antineoplastics cause interference with nucleic acid synthesis by binding to base pairs of DNA and inercalating between adjoining base pairs in the DNA helix structure; DNA-directed RNA and DNA transcription is prevented. The drug is maximally toxic in the S phase of the cell cycle though usually classified as non-cell-cycle-phase specific [36].

The vast majority of experience with the use of doxorubicin instillations into the bladder as therapy for superficial tumors has been gained in Europe and Japan [73−75]. The reported results from use of this agent have been inconsistent. The European investigators do, however, consider doxorubicin to be as effective as thiotepa and significantly less toxic. Table 9 demonstrates the variable nature of the response rates of superficial bladder tumors to doxorubicin. The compilation of European and Japanese data on doxorubicin effectiveness is similar to that described earlier for thiotepa (Table 5): Approximately one-third of patients achieve a complete remission, one-third achieve a partial regression, and the remainig one-third do not respond to therapy. One must remember to keep in mind the heterogeneity of dosing, histology, grade, and other factors that may exist in the superficial bladder population when comparing results of different trials.

Table 9. Doxorubicin response rates in superficial bladder cancer

Author	Patients no.	Complete response no. (%)	Partial response no. (%)	No response no. (%)
Pavone-Macaluso 1971 [132]	5	0 (0)	3 (60)	2 (40)
Ozaki 1977 (see Pavone-Macaluso 1978 [135])	80	22 (27)	35 (44)	23 (29)
Nijima 1978 [125]	194	39 (20)	72 (37)	83 (43)
Edsmyr 1980 [42]	53	37 (70)	5 (9)	11 (21)
Jaske 1981 [75]	15	10 (66)	0 (0)	5 (34)
	347	108 (31)	115 (33)	124 (37)

Niijima [125] possesses the most experience with intravesical doxorubicin. In studying 30-mg, 50-mg, and 60-mg doses given on 3 consecutive days with 2-h retention times, he reported overall response rates of 56%, 72%, and 74%, respectively. No difference in the outcome of therapy was noted when evaluating tumor size or site. Multiple tumors often responded better than solitary types. Niijima also reported results of a collaborative research project conducted in Japan. This study evaluated 194 patients treated three times per week with the previous dose ranges. Results were superior in patients at the 50- and 60-mg doses and in those with multiple tumors. The overall response rates for all three doses were 20% complete (defined as greater than 90% reduction in tumor size), 37% partial, and 43% no responses. Pavone-Macaluso [136] investigated three different doses of doxorubicin instilled into the bladder. He observed no CRs; the partial response rates were 12.5% (2 of 16 patients) with a 10-mg, 30% (three of ten) with a 20-mg, and 33% (one of three) with a 40-mg dose. In contrast, Edsmyr and associates [42] used an 80-mg monthly dose in 58 patients. It was noted that 11 of 11 patients with previously untreated TIS lesions achieved CR on cystoscopy, while 43% (10 of 23) of T1 tumors disappeared. Overall, 70% with TIS or T1 lesions achieved CR and 9% a partial response during therapy as evaluated by cystoscopy. Doxorubicin does appear quite active in carcinoma in situ. Jaske et al. [75] evaluated doses of 40 and 80 mg. There was no significant difference in the remission rates between the two doses. Sixty-six percent (10 of 15) patients achieved a tumor remission, while five patients (33%) failed. Of the failures, only one showed progression over a follow-up period of 6−22 months. Direct injections of doxorubicin into bladder tumors has been reported; however, the results are limited and preliminary in nature [118].

The use of doxorubicin as a prophylactic agent has been explored only by a handful of investigators, often not in well-controlled conditions. Although firm comparisons of doxorubicin with thiotepa are difficult to make due to the frequent lack of control groups and studies of a randomized nature, data thus far suggests that doxorubicin has merit as a prophylactic agent and should be implemented in well-controlled, randomized studies with other agents such as VM-26, thiotepa, and mitomycin-C. Banks et al. [7] found 38% (5 of 13) of patients had tumor recurrence when treated with monthly instillations of doxorubicin with follow-up times up to 21 months. In all patients, the number of recurrent sites decreased. The median range of remission was 10 months, with two of eight responding patients tumor-free at 21 months. Jacobi's group [69] instilled doxorubicin into the bladder 3–4 weeks post-TUR with a 40-mg dose. The mean follow-up time was 22 months (range 16–27). Five of 15 patients (33%) recurred while on treatment. In two patients there was tumor progression, and in two patients recurrences were multifocal. In comparison, 13 of 15 patients in the control group recurred, with four demonstrating tumor progression and ten (77%) showing multifocal recurrences. Schulman et al. [155] administered 50 mg of doxorubicin within 24 h of TUR for T1 bladder tumors according to the following schedule: Twice during week 1, weekly for 4 weeks, thereafter monthly doses. Of the 82 patients treated, 32 (39%) presented with one or more recurrences, 27 of which were T1 lesions; of these, five were more invasive tumors. Of 23 de novo patients, 19 (38%) were free of tumor; of previously treated patients 47% (28 of 59) showed recurrence. The results do not differ significantly from the thiotepa study performed by the National Bladder Cancer Cooperative Group [123]. Jacobi et al. [71] performed a randomized trial comparing VM-26 (50 mg), doxorubicin (50 mg), and mitomycin-C (10 mg), which were administered 4 weeks subsequent to TUR every 2 weeks. Patients were Stage O–A and grades I–III. The follow-up time averaged 11 months (range 9–19). Recurrence-free rates following treatment (6 months) were 81% (doxorubicin), 76% (mitomycin-C), and 81% (VM-26). At the end of the follow-up period, the results were 73%, 74%, and 75%, respectively, with overall recurrence-free rates of 56%, 69%, and 56%. Progressive recurrences (stage or grade) were noted in 17%. Neither multiplicity nor stage proved to be critical factors; however, higher grades were associated within increased recurrence rates (I = 17 and 20%, II = 73 and 57%) for each observation time. It was concluded that all three drugs appeared to be equally efficacious, that low-grade lesions responded better to prophylactic therapy, and the recurrence rates increase with discontinuation of effective therapeutic prophylaxis. It is of note that the dose of mitomycin-C at 10 mg is lower than the traditionally used doses of 20–60 mg. Horn et al. [67] initiated a controlled trial evaluating the prophylactic efficacy of thiotepa versus doxorubicin. Sixty-milligram doses of thiotepa and 50-mg doses of doxorubicin were each given every 3 weeks. Three patients at the beginning of the trial had stage B1 disease. The treatment group in which they were entered was not delineated. After 36 months, cystoscopic evaluation showed only six patients to be in each group, and 14.3% of the doxorubicin patients had recurrent tumors as against 25% of the thiotepa patients. However, the significance of these findings is difficult to interpret, as the patient group size was small and follow-up times were short. The authors plan to continue the protocol over a longer time span so as to evaluate the final efficacy of these two agents on recurrence rate and long-term disease-free period.

Doxorubicin is administered in a similar fashion to the other intravesical chemotherapeutic agents. Following passage of a urethral catheter, the drug is instilled into the bladder, and the patient retains the medication for 2 h before voiding. The most common dose schedules employed are 40–80 mg at a 2-mg/ml concentration given every 3–4 weeks [42, 67, 75, 132]. Most investigators wait 3–4 weeks after TUR and/or fulguration before instilling the drug, as significant systemic absorption may occur (Table 4).

Toxicity of doxorubicin is minimal in comparison to thiotepa. Perhaps this is due to its higher mw (580 and 189, respectively). Although absorption may be significant [134], most investigators [70, 94] have found little systemic absorption of this agent from the bladder. This is supported by the clinical studies carried out thus far; leukopenia has not been reported, and only one case of thrombocytopenia with ECG changes has

Table 10. Doxorubicin as prophylaxis

Author	Patients no.	% Recurrence		Follow-up time (months)
		Control (%)	Treated (%)	
Banks 1977 [7]	13	–	38	21
Jacobi 1978 [69]	30	87	33	22
Schulman 1981 [155]	82	–	39	12 +
Jacobi 1981 [71]	64	–	44	11 (9–19)
Horn 1981 [67]	12	25[a]	14	9

[a] Control group = thiotepa treated

been observed [125]. The most common side effects occur locally. Approximately 30% of patients complain of urgency [125], 5% of which may require discontinuation of therapy [42]. Twenty-six percent of patients have mild local irritative symptoms [155], with about 25% of patients developing chemical cystitis [71, 75, 136, 155]. Urinary tract infection may occur in 15%–30% of patients [69, 75]. Only two cases of hematuria have been reported during therapy [75, 136]. Overall, the toxicologic spectrum of doxorubicin appears similar to that of mitomycin-C and significantly less than that of thiotepa.

Doxorubicin (Adriamycin, Adria Laboratories) is available as 10-mg and 50-mg vials at a cost of $ 16.05 and $ 76.15, respectively. This corresponds to approximately $ 64 per 40-mg, $ 76 per 50-mg, $ 93 per 60-mg, and $ 124 per 80-mg dose [6]. The intact vials may be stored at room temperature prior to use. Normal saline or sterile water for irrigation may be used as diluents in preparing intravesical doses. Following reconstitution, the solutions are stable for 24 h at room temperature and 48 h if refrigerated. Doxorubicin is physically incompatible with a number of agents such as 5-fluorouracil and dexamethasone [36].

Teniposide (VM-26)

Teniposide (VM-26, epipodophyllotoxin) is an investigational chemotherapeutic agent currently being studied in the United States. It is a semisynthetic podophyllin derivative (MW = 656) and possesses poor water-solubility. In systemic use, its antitumor spectrum includes leukemias, Hodgkin's lymphoma, non-Hodgkin's lymphomas, brain neoplasms, and bladder cancers [149]. VM-26 produces its cytotoxic action by binding to microtubular proteins, which arrests cells in the metaphase portion of the cell cycle and therefore inhibits mitosis. Cellular respiration is also impaired at the mitochondrial-electron transport level, thus blocking production of cellular energy [149]. In an animal model, Soloway [161] was able to demonstrate the ability of VM-26 to reduce significantly the incidence of subsequent tumors secondary to implantation. In humans, Pavone-Macaluso [136] was able to demonstrate an overall response rate in 50% (three of six) of patients receiving intravesical VM-26 for superficial bladder tumors. Of these six cases, there were two CRs and one partial response. The two complete responders had multiple recurrent papillomata prior to therapy. Both patients remained tumor-free for over 1 year. Jacobi and associates [71] more recently reported a randomized prophylaxis study of 122 patients treated with intravesical doxorubicin, mitomycin-C, or VM-26. The dose of VM-26 employed was 50 mg/30 ml with instillations beginning 4 weeks following TUR and repeated every 2 weeks for 6 months. Recurrence-free rates were 81% at the end of therapy (6 months) and 56% at the end of the follow-up period (average 11 months). VM-26 was equally effective as doxorubicin or mitomycin-C. In contrast, Soloway [163], in reviewing the EORTC cooperative group study, found that VM-26 provided no significant reduction in recurrences when used as prophylaxis after surgical resection. As with doxorubicin, further evaluation of VM-26 is justified in light of the results, albeit disparate findings, both as definitive therapy and as a prophylactic modality.

VM-26 has a high mw as compared to thiotepa (656 and 189, respectively), and one would not expect a large amount of systemic absorption on this basis. However, due to the lipid-solubility of this agent and its ability to gain entry to the central nervous system and exert activity on cerebral tumors, one would have to be cautious of excluding systemic side effects. With parenteral systemic therapy, toxicity frequently includes a dose-limiting factor of leukopenia and less frequently thrombocytopenia, stomatitis, nausea, vomiting, and alopecia. Acute allergic manifestations may develop with VM-26 and include anaphylactoid reactions, fever, cardiovascular collapse, and respiratory symptoms. Immune depression appears to be minimal [149]. In the limited experience with VM-26 as an intravesical agent, there appears to be minimal systemic absorption from the bladder. Jacobi and associates [71] observed no incidence of systemic toxicity in 16 patients treated with intravesical doses of 50 mg every 2 weeks. The most frequent side effect with VM-26 bladder instillations is chemical cystitis, which required interruption in the therapy of two to six patients in the series of Pavonne-Macaluso and Ingaugiola [136].

VM-26 is administered intravesically as a 50-mg dose in normal saline. The drug is available on an investigational basis in the United States from the National Cancer Institute and is not commercially available. VM-26 is supplied as 50-mg/5-ml ampules. The ampules should be stored at room temperature and protected from light prior to use. When diluted to 30–100 ml with normal saline for bladder instillations, the drug is stable for 4 h at room temperature [120].

Bacillus Calmette-Guerin (BCG)

Immunotherapy may be either specific or nonspecific. Specific immunotherapy has been attempted in bladder cancer by using such modalities as sensitized lymphocytes. The use of nonspecific immunotherapy such as BCG is more widely used and is based in part on the hypothesis that placing an immune stimulant in contact with superficial bladder cells bearing antigenic properties would stimulate a host response to the tumor cells, thus producing a cytotoxic response and a lessening chance of neoplastic transformation. Tumor-specific antigens have been found on the surface of transitional tumor cells [17]. In experimental bladder tumor models, Lamm et al. [88] were able to demonstrate the prevention of bladder tumor progression with intralesional injections of BCG.

Morales and associates [113] in 1976 treated nine patients with combined intradermal and intravesical BCG to prevent recurrence or ablate residual tumor. Four of nine patients responded to therapy. One patient with persistent tumor achieved CR with no recurrences for 20 months. The remaining three responders had no recurrence during follow-up times of 22 weeks, 6 months, and 13 months. Post-BCG recurrence rates were significantly less than pretreatment. Martinez-Pineiro and Muntanola [101] administered intralesional injections into bladder tumors of two patients and noted regressions in both. One of the patients, however, experienced a severe hypersensitivity reaction. A later follow-up [112] of the earlier report by Morales et al. [113] found a significant reduction in the recurrence rate in 16 patients as compared to pretreatment statistics (seven recurrences per 222 treated patient-months versus 53 recurrences per 162 nontreated patient-months; $p < 0.05$). Douville et al. [37] applied BCG by abdominal scarification and intravesical instillation. Four of six patients responded completely to this therapy, however two patients experienced major systemic complications requiring antitubercular drugs. Impressive results have been reported with carcinoma in situ in one small study. Morales [114] treated seven carcinoma in situ patients with intradermal and intravesical BCG. Five of seven patients (71%) achieved tumor-free status for periods ranging from 12 to 33 months (mean 22.6).

Winters and Lamm [189] treated 60 patients utilizing the same regimen as described by Morales [114] and Morales et al. [113]. Following randomization, 21% (6 of 29) of BCG-therapy patients had tumor recurrence as against 46% (13 of 28) of the nontreated group. The mean disease-free interval for the BCG versus the nontreated group was significantly different (23.6 months versus 14.7 months). Average time up to recurrence for the BCG group was 8.2 months and for the nontreated group 7.6 months. Purified protein derivative (PPD) skin test correlated with BCG antibody levels as an immune indicator in only 14 of 27 BCG therapy patients. Other findings suggested that decreasing antibody response to BCG paralleled an increased risk of tumor recurrence in treatment patients. More recently, Morales et al. [115] treated 17 patients with incompletely resected transitional cell tumors of the bladder with BCG. Ten patients (59%) had complete ablation of tumors and remained tumor-free for the follow-up period (12−30 months). The mean interval free of disease was 19.1 months. These initial results merit further investigation of the intravesical use of BCG both for the therapy and prophylaxis of superficial bladder cancer in larger prospective randomized trials against other chemotherapeutic agents and in combination with other agents. It would also be of interest to define whether the effect of BCG is a local inflammation or is a true immunologic response.

The usual method of treatment with BCG is by a combined administration of intradermal and intravesical instillation. The usual BCG dose is 5 mg intradermally into the upper thigh (alternating sides) and instillation of 120 mg in 50 ml normal saline into the bladder utilizing a 2-h retention time [113]. The patient should change positions every 15 min to ensure complete bladder contact with the drug [115]. Treatment is repeated for a total of 6 consecutive weeks.

Side effects during BCG therapy are very common but are usually mild in nature. Most patients complain of irritative symptoms with up to a 90% rate of dysuria and frequency [89]. About 40% of patients have hematuria [89] and 20%−40% may experience a low-grade fever, which generally resolves in 1−2 days [89, 112, 114, 115]. Hypersensitivity reactions have been noted in two of four patients in one study [37]. Three patients have had major systemic complications which necessitated treatment with antitubercular agents [37, 115]. A number of patients may also complain of flu-like symptoms [115]. Although the side effects to BCG are common, the symptoms are generally mild, and in very few patients was it necessary to discontinue therapy or interrupt the therapeutic schedules.

Other Pharmacologic Therapies

Pyridoxine (Vitamin B_6) has recently been studied as a prophylactic regimen for decreasing recurrences that theoretically occur from the continued presence of tumor-inducing or -promoting substances in the urine. Animal studies have indicated that tryptophan metabolites produce bladder cancer in mice [16]. Yoshida et al. [191] studied tryptophan metabolism in patients with low-stage bladder cancer. Over a 5-year follow-up period, all of the patients with abnormal tryptophan metabolism had recurrences, whereas only 60% of patients with normal tryptophan metabolism had tumor recurrences over the same period. Byar and Blackard [19] reported a study by Brown's group [16] which demonstrated that daily doses of 25 mg oral pyridoxine given to patients with abnormal tryptophan metabolites would restore urinary levels to normal. It is thought that 50% of patients with bladder cancer have abnormal tryptophan metabolism. In randomizing 121 patients for placebo, pyridoxine, or intravesical thiotepa, Byar's group found that pyridoxine significantly lowered tumor recurrence rate, as compared to controls, if patients who had recurrences during the first 10 months, or who were followed-up for less than 10 months were excluded ($p = 0.03$).

Another pharmacologic therapy of interest, although not a mode of intravesical chemotherapy, is that of chemoprevention with synthetic analogs of vitamin A (retinoids). In theory, chemoprevention during the preneoplastic phase is an attempt at reversing the progression of premalignant cells to invasive malignancy by noncytotoxic physiologic mechanisms. Retinoids are potent agents in the control of maturation and cell differentiation of many epithelial tissues, including the bladder. Biochemically, retinoids play a critical role in DNA synthesis and mitotic activity in epithelia. Organ cultures of prostate glands have shown the ability of retinoids to reverse the pathologic lesions induced by chemical carcinogens [166]. Retinoid deficiency has been demonstrated to enhance the susceptibility of experimental animal bladders to chemical carcinogenesis [24]. 13-cis-retinoic acid is a synthetic retinoid analog undergoing clinical trials because this agent is less toxic than trans-retinoic acid and, in contrast to retinyl esters, is neither stored in the liver nor transported in the blood by retinol binding protein [167]. In animal studies with oral dosing, 13-cis-retinoic acid is able to inhibit the incidence, number, and severity of bladder cancers, even if chemoprevention is begun after completion of carcinogen treatment [10, 167, 168]. In these animal models, 13-cis-retinoic acid was able to cause significant inhibition of both preneoplastic and neoplastic lesions in the bladder [10, 168]. The number of studies in humans has been minimal. Peck and Yoder [137] found significant activity of 13-cis-retinoic acid in keratinizing dermatoses. The starting dose was 1 mg/kg/day increasing by 2−3 week intervals until therapeutic benefit or toxicity was observed. Toxicity was minimal with 69% (9 of 13) of patients experiencing cheilitis, which was controlled with petrolatum, 15% (2 of 15) developed symptoms of dry nasal mucosa, and one patient, after discontinuing therapy at a dose of 2 mg/kg/day with complaints of irritation in the eyes, blurred vision, arthralgias, and perioral dermatitis, had his symptoms cleared within 2 weeks. Kerr and associates [81] studied the clinical pharmacology of this retinoid with oral doses of 0.5 mg/kg/day escalating to 8 mg/kg/day over 4 weeks. All patients experienced toxicity (unspecified) after 4 weeks. Based on measured serum levels and previous in vitro data, the investigators concluded that this dose schedule may not be optimal to control neoplastic growth. Presant et al. [139] studied 13-cis-retinoic acid in four chronic granulocytic leukemia patients randomized with and without busulfan. The dose of retinoid used was 2 mg/kg/day. All four patients receiving retinoic acid experienced dose-limiting skin toxicity consisting of dryness in two, erythema in two, and desquamation in three patients. One patient had conjunctivitis, two had hypertryglyceridemia ($> 50\%$ more than pretreatment), and two had serum glutamic-oxaloacetic transaminase (SGOT) elevations ($> 50\%$ more than pretreatment). The investigators concluded that 13-cis-retinoic acid is well tolerated if intermittantly discontinued for recovery from skin, hypertriglyceridemia, or hepatic toxicity. Koontz [83] reported a cooperative pilot study beginning in the United States to assess the chemopreventative efficacy of 13-cis-retinoic acid. Eighty-four patients would have received the drug 2 weeks after the patient was determined to be free of bladder cancer by cystoscopic and cytologic studies. 13-cis-retinoic acid would have been given for 6 months, with cystoscopy every 3 months for a follow-up time of 2 years. The 13-cis-retinoic acid National Bladder Collaborative Group A study was later terminated after 22 patients suffered blepharoconjunctivitis and cutaneous toxicity, as well as a projected lack of efficacy [29].

It is possible that chemoprophylaxis may be achieved by the oral administration of antineoplastic agents. Oral treatment is limited by the low urinary excretion of most active antineoplastic agents. Although the oral route of administration may not be advantageous from the standpoint of systemic toxicity, this route could hypothetically provide cytotoxic concentrations of the drug in the plasma and urine more frequently and for longer periods of time than can be achieved by direct bladder instillations. A drug that could test this hypothesis would be methotrexate. This cell-cycle-specific folate antagonist is well absorbed by the oral route (about 100% in doses < 30 mg/m^2), and its urinary excretion may be approximately 90% over 24 h [12]. Another attractive feature of this drug is that it has shown antitumor activity in locoregional (T2 and T3) and disseminated bladder cancer [56, 119, 171, 190]. Hall and associates [58] tested this hypothesis utilizing methotrexate at a weekly dose of 50 mg in 14 patients as definitive therapy and 17 patients as prophylactic therapy post-TUR. Of the 14 patients receiving definitive therapy, 5 of 14 (36%) achieved a partial remission after 6–16 weeks of treatment and 7 of 17 (41%) of prophylactic therapy patients were free of tumor. Fifty-three percent (9 of 17) had decreased frequency and decreased numbers of recurrences during the average follow-up period of 8.9 months (range 2–19). The treatment was well tolerated. These results merit further evaluation over an extended follow-up period with randomization against intravesically instilled chemotherapy.

Other Nonchemotherapy Treatments

Although the main goal of this paper is to review the intravesical chemotherapy of superficial bladder cancer, nonchemotherapeutic means will be briefly discussed to put the whole therapeutic spectrum of this disease into perspective and to give some insight into possible future multimodality therapies.

Radiotherapy in superficial bladder cancer, when administered prophylactically in low doses, does little to reduce the number or severity of recurrences [131], although it has been shown to improve ureteral obstruction [23]. Results of suprapubic radium needle implantation have been encouraging. The overall mortality has been low, and urinary and sexual functions have been preserved. Experience with this mode of therapy has

Table 11. Comparative response rates of intravesical chemotherapeutic agents as definitive therapy (Tables 7–9)

Drug	Patients no.	Complete response rate no. (%)	Partial response rate no. (%)	Remissions (CR + PR) no. (%)
Thiotepa	231	88 (38)	56 (24)	144 (62)
Epodyl	279	126 (45)	71 (25)	197 (70)
Mitomycin-C	187	108 (58)	33 (18)	141 (76)
Doxorubicin	347	108 (31)	115 (33)	223 (64)

Table 12. Recommended patient care in intravesical chemotherapy

1. Prior to therapy, the following laboratory tests should be performed:
   a) White blood cell count: should be greater than $3,500/mm^3$
   b) Platelet count: should be greater than $100,000/mm^3$
   c) Red blood cell count
   d) Hemoglobin
   e) Hematocrit (packed cell volume)
   f) Urinalysis
   g) Urine cytology.

2. The patient should be monitored for signs and symptoms of urinary infection (e.g., painful urination, frequency, cloudy urine, hematuria)

3. The patient should refrain from fluid intake for 8–12 h prior to therapy and during the 2-h instillation period to prevent excessive diuresis and facilitate retention of the medication in the bladder for the prescribed time period

4. During retention of the instilled drug, the patient should be observed for allergic drug reactions, especially with agents such as BCG

5. After voiding the medication, the patient should wash his/her hands and perineal area thoroughly to aid in preventing contact dermatitis. Should palmar rash occur, this may respond to topical corticosteroid therapy

6. Prophylactic antimicrobial agents may be considered in patients who develop chronic or frequent urinary infections (e.g., sulfamethoxazole, cotrimoxazole, ampicillin). Most cases of infection appear to be coliform bacteria

7. Patients should void as frequently as possible after therapy, as residual drug in bladder may exacerbate or induce chemical cystitis

only been obtained by Van der Werf-Messing and Hop at the Rotterdam Radiotherapy Institute [176–178]. Three hundred and forty-five T1 patients were separated in a nonrandomized fashion, 148 patients receiving TUR alone and 197 patients receiving TUR plus radium implants. In the TUR group, 75% had at least one relapse compared with 18% in the radium group. Of the radium group 80% were relapse-free after 5 years versus 20% for the TUR only group. It would be of interest to see if these results could be duplicated in other institutions in a prospective randomized trial.

Botto et al. [13] have reported good results in treating primarily T1 tumors with iridium-192, in an uncontrolled study. In the first 3 years of follow-up, 2 of 17 (12%) patients had tumor recurrence. Further study of this procedure is warranted. Uyama and associates [175] produced encouraging results with the combination of intravesical doxorubicin combined with low-dose irradiation (800 rad) in a small group of patients with low-grade superficial bladder cancer. In ten patients receiving this combined modality therapy, there were three complete responses and six partial responses on cystoscopy. Further study by this group found a complete response rate of 10% in 49 patients treated doxorubicin alone versus 18% in 49 patients treated with a combination of doxorubicin plus radiation, when evaluated by cystoscopy. These results warrant further evaluation of this combined modality in a larger patient population. Further experience is required to define the exact role of other modalities such as Helmstein's distension [46], hyperthermia [57], and hydrostatic pressure [63].

Future Prospects and Conclusion

Management of the superficial bladder cancer patient consists of two complementary but separate therapeutic goals: Treatment of the existing tumor(s) and prevention of tumor recurrence. At present, the stage, grade, and multicentricity are the major determinants in the natural and therapeutic history of the disease. Although intravesical instillation of chemotherapeutic agents has been employed for 20 or so years, neither its exact role nor the optimal dose, schedule of administration, and potential carcinogenic effects have been established. To date, dramatic differences in efficacy between the agents commonly used for intravesical chemotherapy, either as definitive therapy or prophylaxis, have not been appreciated. These agents do appear to lower the recurrence rate as well as extend the disease-free survival time. Thiotepa is the agent that other agents should be compared with from both an efficacy standpoint and a toxicologic evaluation.

Different administration schedules and modalities alone or in combination need further study, such as the utility of continuous bladder irrigation, the use of sequential chemotherapeutic agents to gain cell synchronization, and the use of multiple drug regimens. As there are multiple factors that influence the occurrence and history of bladder cancer, multimodality therapy deserves testing. Such modes of therapy that could be used together to act by a different mechanism or on a different factor would be intravesical chemotherapy with cytotoxic agents, radioactive needle implants, carcinogen modifiers such as pyridoxine, chemoprotective agents such as retinoic acid, and immune stimulants such as BCG. These studies should be performed in a randomized prospective controlled fashion, which may require cooperative multiinstitutional involvement to accrue adequate numbers of patients.

At this time there are a number of important questions that remain to be answered concerning the treatment of superficial bladder cancer: 1) does this mode of therapy affect overall long-term survival? 2) does prophylactic intravesical chemotherapy alter the incidence of subsequent invasive disease? 3) does intravesical chemotherapy alter the sites, incidence, or responsiveness of subsequent metastatic disease? 4) and what is the optimal duration of prophylactic therapy from a cost-effectiveness standpoint? We expect that these promising areas and questions in the treatment of superficial bladder cancer will be subjects of future investigations in this area.

References

1. Abassian A, Wallace DM (1966) Intracavitary chemotherapy of diffuse non-infiltrating papillary carcinoma of the bladder. J Urol 96: 461
2. Allen TD, Henderson BW (1965) Adenocarcinoma of the bladder. J Urol 93: 50−56
3. Althausen AF, Prout GR, Daly JJ (1976) Non-invasive papillary carcinoma of the bladder associated with carcinoma in situ. J Urol 116: 575
4. American Cancer Society (1982) Cancer Facts and Figures (1981). American Cancer Society, New York
5. American Cancer Society (1980) Cancer statistics. Cancer 30: 24
6. American Druggist Blue Book (July 1981 − June 1982). Hearst, New York
7. Banks MD, Pontes JE, Izbicki RM, Pierce JM (1977) Topical instillation of doxorubicin hydrochloride in the treatment of recurring superficial transitional cell carcinoma of the bladder. J Urol 118: 757−760
8. Barnes RW, Bergman RT, Hadley HL, Jonston OL (1967) Control of bladder tumors by endoscopic surgery. J Urol 97: 864
9. Barnes RW, Dick AL, Hadley HL, Johnston OL (1977) Survival following transurethral resection of bladder carcinoma. Cancer Res 37: 2895−2897
10. Becci PJ, Thompson HJ, Grubbs CJ, Brown CC, Moon RC (1979) Effect of delay in administration of 13-cis retinoic acid on the inhibition of urinary bladder carcinogenesis in the rat. Cancer Res 39: 3141−3144
11. Bessman JD, Johnson RK, Goldin A (1975) Permeability of normal and cancerous rat bladder to antineoplastic agents. Urology 6: 187−193
12. Bleyer WA (1977) Methotrexate: clinical pharmacology, current status and therapeutic guidelines. Cancer Treat Rev 4: 87−101
13. Botto H, Perrin JL, Auvert J, Salle M, Pierquin B (1980) Treatment of malignant bladder tumors by iridium-192 wiring. Urology 16: 467−469
14. Bracken RB, Johnson DE, Rodriguez L, Samuels ML, Ayala A (1977) Treatment of multiple superficial tumors of bladder with intravesical bleomycin. Urology 9: 161−163
15. Broders AC (1922) Epithelioma of the genitourinary organs. Ann Surg 75: 574
16. Brown RR, Price JM, Sutter EJ, Wear JB (1960) The metabolism of tryptophan in patients with bladder cancer. Cancer Res 16: 299
17. Bubenik J, Peremann P, Helmstain K, Moberger G (1970) Cellular and humoral immune responses to human urinary bladder carcinomas. Int J Cancer 5: 310
18. Burnand KG, Boyd PJR, Mayo ME, Shuttleworth KED, Lloyd-Davies RW (1976) Intravesical thiotepa as an adjuvant to cystodiathermy in the treatment of transitional cell bladder cancer. Br J Urol 48: 55−59
19. Byar D, Blackard C (1977) Comparisons of placebo, pyridoxine, and topical thiotepa in preventing recurrence of Stage 1 bladder cancer. Urology 10: 556−561
20. Camuzzi F, Bondhus M, Lockhart J, Politano V (1980) Mitomycin-C in the treatment of superficial bladder cancer. Am Urol Assn Proc, Abstract 120
21. Case RAM, Hosker ME, McDonald DB, Pearson JT (1954) Tumors of the urinary bladder in workmen engaged in the manufacture and use of certain dye stuffs intermediates in the British chemical industry. The role of aniline, benzidine, alpha-naphthylamine, and beta-naphthylamine. Br J Ind Med 11: 75
22. Case RAM, Hosker ME (1954) Tumor of the urinary bladder as an occupational disease in the rubber industry in England and Wales. Br J Prev Soc Med 8: 39−50
23. Chan RC, Bracken RB, Johnson DE (1979) Single dose whole pelvis megavoltage irradiation for palliative control of hematuria or ureteral obstruction. J Urol 122: 750−751
24. Cohen SM, Wittenberg JF, Bryan GT (1974) Effect of hyper- and avitaminosis A on urinary bladder carcinogenicity of N-(4-(5-nitro-2-furyl)-2-thiazolyl)-formamide (FANT). Fed Proc 33: 602

25. Cole P, Hoover R, Friedell GH (1972) Occupation and cancer of the lower urinary tract. Cancer 29: 1250
26. Colleen S, Ek A, Hellsten S, Lindholm CE (1980) Intracavitary Epodyl for multiple, non-invasive highly differentiated bladder tumors. Scand J Urol Nephrol 14: 43–45
27. Connolly JG, Anderson C, Johnson I (1979) Some newer approaches to the treatment of the mucosa of patients with superficial bladder cancer: 1. Continuous bladder irrigation with 5-fluorouracil. Can Med Assoc J 121: 318–320
28. Cooper PH, Waisman J, Johnston WH, Skinner DG (1973) Severe atypia of transitional epithelium and carcinoma of the urinary bladder. Cancer 31: 1055
29. Corder MP, Stamp DC (1982) Chemotherapeutic approaches to transitional cell carcinoma of the bladder: part 1, superficial disease; chemoprevention. In: Bonney WW, Prout GR (eds) AUA Monographs, vol 1, bladder cancer. Williams and Wilkins, Baltimore, pp 165–172
30. Cox CE, Cass AS, Boyce WH (1968) Bladder cancer: a 26 year review. Trans Am Assoc Genitourin Surg 60: 22–30
31. Day JW, Shrivastav S, Lin G, Bonar RA, Paulson DF (1981) In vitro chemotherapeutic testing of urologic tumors. J Urol 125: 490–492
32. De Furia MD, Bracken RB, Johnson DE, Soloway MS, Merrin LE, Morgan LR, Miller HC, Crooke ST (1980) Phase I–II study of Mitomycin C topical therapy for low grade, low stage transitional cell carcinoma of the bladder: an interim report. Cancer Treat Rep 64: 225–230
33. Dean AC, Mostofi FK, Thomason RV, Clark ML (1954) A restudy of the first 1400 tumors in the bladder tumor registry. AFIP J Urol 71: 571–590
34. Denning CL (1950) The biological behavior of transitional cell papilloma of the bladder. J Urol 63: 815–819
35. Dickson RJ, Lang EK (1960) Treatment of papillomata of the bladder with radioactive colloidal gold (Au^{198}) Am J Roentgen 83: 116
36. Dorr RT, Fritz WL (1980) Cancer chemotherapy handbook. Elsevier-Holland, New York
37. Douville Y, Pelouze G, Roy R, Charrois R, Kibrite A, Martin M, Dionne L, Coulonval L, Robinson J (1978) Recurrent bladder papillomata treated with bacillus Calmette-Guerin: a preliminary report. Cancer Treat Rep 62: 551
38. Drew JE, Marshall VF (1968) The effects of topical thiotepa on the recurrence rate of superficial bladder cancer. J Urol 99: 740–743
39. Duckworth DA (1950) The treatment of papillomatosis with podophyllin. J Urol 64: 740
40. Durrant KR, Laing AH (1975) Treatment of multiple superficial papillary tumors of the bladder by intracavitary Yttrium-99. J Urol 113: 480–482
41. Edsmyr F, Boman J (1970) Instillation of thiotepa in vesical papillomatosis. Acta Radiol [Ther] (Stockh) 9: 395–400
42. Edsmyr F, Berlin T, Boman J, Duchek M, Eposti PL, Gustafsson H, Wijkstrom H, Collste LG (1980) Intravesical therapy with adriamycin in patients with superficial bladder tumors. Eur Urol 6: 132–136
43. Einhorn J, Hultzberg S, Nilson A (1964) Treatment of papillomatosis of the bladder with radioactive arsenic ^{76}As. Acta Radiol Ther 2: 1–16
44. Eisenberg RB, Roth RB, Schweinsberg MH (1960) Bladder tumors and associated proliferative mucosal lesions. J Urol 84: 544
45. Eksborg S, Nilsson S, Edsmyr F (1980) Intravesical instillation of adriamycin: a model for standardization of the chemotherapy. Eur Urol 6: 218–220
46. England HR, Rigby C, Shepheard BGF, Tresidder GC, Blandy JP (1973) Evaluation of Helmstein's distension method for carcinoma of the bladder. Br J Urol 45: 593
47. Esquivel EL, MacKenzie R, Whitmore WF (1965) Treatment of bladder tumors by instillation of thiotepa, actinomycin D, or 5-fluorouracil. Invest Urol 2: 381–386

48. Farrow GM, Utz DC, Rite CC (1976) Morphological and clinical observations of patients with early bladder cancer treated with total cystectomy. Cancer Res 36:2495

49. Farrow GM, Utz DC, Rite CC, Greene LF (1977) Clinical observation on 69 cases of in situ carcinoma of the urinary bladder. Cancer Res 37:2794−2798

50. Fitzpatrick JM, Khan O, Oliver RTD, Riddle PR (1979) Long term follow-up in patients with superficial bladder tumors treated with intravesical Epodyl. Br J Urol 51:545−548

51. Flocks RH (1951) Treatment of patients with carcinoma of the bladder. JAMA 145:295−301

52. Franksson C (1950) Tumors of the urinary bladder: a pathological and clinical study of 434 cases. ACTA Chir Scand [Suppl] 515:1−203

53. Gavrell GJ, Lewis RW, Meehan WL, Leblanc GA (1978) Intravesical thiotepa in the immediate postoperative period in patients with recurrent transitional cell carcinoma of the bladder, J Urol 120:410−411

54. Gowing NFC (1960) Urethral carcinoma associated with cancer of the bladder. Br J Urol 32:428−439

55. Greene LF, Hanash KA, Farrow GM (1973) Benign papilloma or papillary carcinoma of the bladder? J Urol 110:205

56. Hall RR, Bloom HJG, Freeman JE, Nawrocki A, Wallace DM (1974) Methotrexate treatment for advanced bladder cancer. Br J Urol 46:431−438

57. Hall RR, Shade RO, Swinney J (1974) Effects of hyperthermia on bladder cancer. Br Med J 2:593−594

58. Hall RR, Herring DW, McGill AC, Gibb I (1981) Oral methotrexate therapy for multiple superficial bladder carcinomata. Cancer Treat Rep 65 (Suppl 1):175−178

59. Hendry WF, Gowing NFC, Wallace DM (1974) Surgical treatment of urethral tumors associated with bladder cancer. Proc R Soc Med 67:304

60. Herring HT (1903) The treatment of vesical papilloma by injections. Br Med J 2:1398

61. Hicks RM (1966) The permeability of rat transitional cell epithelium. J Cell Biol 28:21

62. Hinman F (1956) Recurrence of bladder tumors by surgical implantation. J Urol 75:695−696

63. Hirose K, Seto T, Takayasu H (1977) Re-evaluation of hydrostatic pressure treatment for malignant bladder lesions. J Urol 118:762

64. Hisazumi H, Uchibayashi T, Naito K, Misaki T, Miyazaki K (1975) The prophylactic use of thiotepa and urokinase in transitional cell carcinoma of the bladder: a preliminary report. J Urol 114:394

65. Hollands FG (1950) The results of diathermy treatment of villous papilloma of the bladder. Br J Urol 22:342−375

66. Hollister D, Coleman M (1980) Hematologic effects of intravesicular thiotepa therapy for bladder carcinoma. JAMA 244:2065−2067

67. Horn Y, Eidelman A, Walach N, Ilian M (1981) Intravesical chemotherapy in a controlled trial with thiotepa versus doxorubicin hydrochloride. J Urol 125:652−654

68. Issel BF, DeFuria MD, Fandrich SE (1981) Topical mitomycin-C in thiotepa refractory non-invasive bladder cancer. Am Soc Clin Oncol Proc 22:464

69. Jacobi GH, Kurth KH, Klippel KF, Hohenfellner R (1978) On the biological behavior of T2 transitional cell tumors of the urinary bladder and initial results of the prophylactic use of topical adriamycin under controlled and randomized conditions. In: WHO, Diagnostics and treatment of superficial urinary bladder tumors. Collaborating centre for research and treatment of bladder cancer, Stockholm, pp 83−94

70. Jacobi GH, Kurth K (1980) Studies on the intravesical action of topically administered G^3H-doxorubicin hydrochloride in men: plasma uptake and tumor penetration. J Urol 124:34−37

71. Jacobi GH, Jaske G, Thuroff JW, Bauer HW (1981) Intravesical chemotherapy for prophylaxis of recurrent superficial bladder tumors: a randomized trial of 122 patients. Am Urol Assn Meeting Abstract 579

72. Jacobo E, Loening S, Schmidt JD, Culp DA (1977) Primary adenocarcinoma of the bladder: a retrospective study of 20 patients. J Urol 117: 54−56

73. Jaske G, Hofstadter F (1980) Intravesical doxorubicin hydrochloride in the management of carcinoma in situ of the bladder. Eur Urol 6: 103−106

74. Jaske G (1981) Intracavitary doxorubicin hydrochloride treatment for carcinoma in situ of the urinary bladder. Eur Urol 7: 68−72

75. Jaske G, Hofstadter F, Marberger H (1981) Intracavitary doxorubicin hydrochloride therapy for carcinoma in situ of the bladder. J Urol 125: 185−189

76. Jewett HJ, Strong GH (1946) Infiltrating carcinoma of the bladder. Relation of depth of penetration of the bladder wall to incidence of local extension and metastasis. J Urol 55: 366

77. Johnson DE, Schaenwald MB, Ayala AG, Miller LS (1976) Squamous cell carcinoma of the bladder. J Urol 115: 542−544

78. Jones HC, Swinney J (1961) Thiotepa in the treatment of tumors of the bladder. Lancet 2: 615

79. Joseph E (1919) Eine neue Methode zur Behandlung der Blasengeschwulste, vorläufige Mitteilung. Zentralbl Chir 46: 931

80. Kaufman JJ, Walthur PJ, Smith RB, Skinner DG (1979) Intracavitary Mitomycin-C in the treatment of superficial urothelial tumors: a preliminary report. Trans Am Assoc Genitourin Surg 71: 6−7

81. Kerr IG, Lippman M, Jenkins J, Meyers C (1981) Clinical pharmacology of 13-cis-retinoic acid. Proc Am Soc Clin Oncol 22: 357 Abstract

82. Keiter JH (1953) Bladder tumor recurrences in the urethra: a warning. J Urol 60: 652−656

83. Koontz WW (1979) Intravesical chemotherapy and chemoprevention of superficial, low grade, low stage bladder carcinoma. Semin Oncol 6: 217−219

84. Koontz WW, Prout GR, Smith W, Frable WJ, Minnis JE (1981) The use of intravesical thiotepa in the management of non-invasive carcinoma of the bladder. J Urol 125: 307−312

85. Koss LG, Melamed MR, Kelly RE (1969) Further cytologic and histologic studies of bladder lesions in workers exposed to para-aminodiphenyl: progress report. J Natl Cancer Inst 43: 233−243

86. Koss LG (1977) Some ultrastructural aspects of experimental and human carcinoma of the bladder. Cancer Res 37: 2824

87. Koss LG, Tiamson EM, Robbins MA (1974) Mapping cancerous and precancerous bladder changes. A study of the urothelium in ten surgically removed bladders. JAMA 227: 281

88. Lamm DL, Harris SC, Gittes RF (1977) Bacillus Calmette-Guerin and dinitrochlorobenzene immunotherapy of chemically induced bladder tumors. Invest Urol 14: 369

89. Lamm DL, Thor DE, Winters WD, Stogdill VD, Radwin HM (1981) BCG immunotherapy of bladder cancer: inhibition of tumor recurrence and associated immune responses. Cancer 38: 82−88

90. Leissner K, Gustavsson B, Nilsson S, Almersjo O (1978) General resorption of intravesically instilled 5-fluorouracil. J Urol 120: 407−409

91. Lerman RI, Hutter RVP, Whitmore WF (1970) Papilloma of the urinary bladder. Cancer 25: 333−342

92. Lilienfeld AM (1964) The relationship of bladder cancer to smoking. Am J Public Health 54: 1864

93. Loening S, Narayana A, Yoder L, Slyman D, Weinstein S, Penick G, Culp D (1980) Factors influencing the recurrence rate of bladder cancer. J Urol 123: 29

94. Lundbeck F, Pederson D, Stroyer I, Uldall A (1981) Absorption of doxorubicin hydrochloride during bladder washings in treatment of non-invasive bladder tumors. Urology 18: 161−163
95. Lutzeyer W, Rubben H, Dahm H (1982) Prognostic parameters in superficial bladder cancer: an analysis of 315 cases. J Urol 127: 250−252
96. MacKenzie N, Torti FM, Faysal M (1981) The natural history of superficial bladder tumors. Proc Am Assoc Cancer Res 22: 198
97. Maluf NSR (1953) Absorption of water, urea, glucose and electrolytes through the human bladder. J Urol 98: 470
98. Marberger J, Marberger M, Decristoforo A (1972) The current status of transurethral resection in the diagnosis and therapy of carcinoma of the urinary bladder. Int J Urol Nephrol 4: 35−44
99. Marshall VF (1952) The relation of the preoperative estimate to the pathologic demonstration of the extent of vesical neoplasm. J Urol 68: 714
100. Wade A, Reynolds JEF (eds) (1977) Martindales: the extra pharmacopia, 27th edn. Pharmaceutical Press, London
101. Martinez-Pineiro JA, Muntanola P (1977) Non-specific immunotherapy with BCG vaccine in bladder tumors: a preliminary report. Eur Urol 3: 11
102. McDonald DF, Thorsen T (1956) Clinical implications of transplantability of induced bladder tumors to intact transitional epithelium in dogs. J Urol 75: 690
103. Melicow MM (1952) Histological study of vesical urothelium intervening between gross neoplasms in total cystectomy. J Urol 68: 261
104. Melicow MM (1955) Tumor of the urinary bladder, a clinicopathological analysis of over 2500 specimens and biopsies. J Urol 74: 498−521
105. Melicow MM (1978) The urothelium: a battleground for oncogenesis. J Urol 120: 43
106. Miller AB (1977) The etiology of bladder cancer from the epidemiological viewpoint. Cancer Res 37: 2939−2942
107. Milner WA (1954) The role of conservative surgery in the treatment of bladder tumors. Br J Urol 26: 375−384
108. Mishina T, Oda K, Murata S, Ooe H, Yasuyuki M, Takahashi T (1975) Mitomycin-C bladder instillation therapy for bladder tumors. J Urol 114: 217−219
109. Mishina T, Watanabe H (1979) Mitomycin-C bladder instillation therapy for bladder tumors. In: Carter SK, Crooke ST (eds) Mitomycin-C: current status and new developments. Academic, New York, pp 193−203
110. Mitchell RJ (1971) Intravesical thiotepa in the treatment of transitional cell bladder carcinoma. Br J Urol 43: 185−188
111. Morales A, Eidinger D, Bruce AW (1976) Intracavitary bacillus Calmette-Guerin in the treatment of superficial bladder tumors. J Urol 116: 180
112. Morales A (1978) Adjuvant immunotherapy in superficial bladder cancer. Natl Cancer Inst Monogr 49: 315−319
113. Morales A, Eidinger D, Bruce AW (1976) Intracavitary bacillus Calmette-Guerin in the treatment of superficial bladder tumors. J Urol 116: 180−183
114. Morales A (1980) Treatment of carcinoma in situ of the bladder with BCG: a phase II trial. Cancer Immunol Immunother 9: 69−72
115. Morales A, Ottenhof P, Emerson L (1981) Treatment of residual, noninfiltrating bladder cancer with bacillus Calmette-Guerin. J Urol 125: 649−651
116. Murphy WM, Soloway MS, Finebaum PJ (1981) Pathological changes associated with topical chemotherapy for superficial bladder cancer. J Urol 126: 461−464
117. Murphy W, Nagy GK, Rao MK, Soloway MS, Parija GC, Cox CE, Friedell GH (1979) Normal urothelium in patients with bladder cancer. Cancer 44: 1050
118. Nakazono M, Iwata S (1978) A preliminary study of chemotherapeutic treatment for bladder tumors. J Urol 119: 598−600
119. Natale RB, Yagoda A, Watson RC, Whitmore WF, Blumenreich M, Braun DW (1981) Methotrexate: an active drug in bladder cancer. Cancer 47: 1246−1250

120. NCI Investigational Drugs: Pharmaceutical Data 1981, Pharmaceutical Resources Branch, Developmental Therapeutics Program, Division of Cancer Treatment, National Cancer Institute, US Dept of Health and Human Services, National Institutes of Health, Washington DC, p 91

121. Needles B, Blumenreich M, Yagoda A, Sogani P, Whitmore WF (1981) Intraversical cisplatin for superficial bladder cancer. Am Assoc Cancer Res 22:158

122. Nichols JA, Marshall VF (1956) Treatment of histologically benign papilloma of the urinary bladder by local excision and fulguration. Cancer 9:566–567

123. Nieh PT, Daly JJ, Heaney JA, Heney NM, Prout GM (1978) The effect of intravesical thiotepa on normal and tumor urothelium. J Urol 119:59–61

124. Nielsen HV, Thybo E (1979) Epodyl treatment of bladder tumors. Scand J Urol Nephrol 13:59–63

125. Niijima T (1978) Intravesical therapy with adriamycin and new trends in the diagnostics and therapy of superficial bladder tumors. In: WHO, Diagnostics and treatment of superficial urinary bladder tumors. Collaborating centre for research and treatment of urinary bladder cancer, Stockholm, pp 37–44

126. Nissenkorn I, Herrod H, Soloway MS (1981) Side effects associated with intravesical Mitomycin-C. J Urol 126:586–587

127. Nocks BN, Nieh PT, Prout GR (1979) A longitudinal study of patients with superficial bladder carcinoma. J Urol 122:27–29

128. O'Flynn JD, Smith M, Hanson JS (1975) Transurethral resection for the assessment and treatment of vesical neoplasms. Eur Urol 1:38–40

129. Olsson CA, DeVere-White RW (1979) Cancer of the bladder In: Javadpour N (ed) Principles and management of urologic cancer. Williams and Wilkins, Baltimore

130. Oravisto KJ (1965) Topical use of thiotepa for tumors of the bladder. Urol Int 20:23–38

131. Page BH, Levison V, Curwen MP (1979) A trial of prophylactic radiotherapy for non-infiltrating bladder tumors. Br J Urol 51:197–199

132. Pavone-Macaluso M (1971) Chemotherapy of vesical and prostatic tumors. Br J Urol 43:701–708

133. Pavone-Macaluso M, Caramia G (1972) Adriamycin and daunomycin in the treatment of vesical and prostatic neoplasias: preliminary results. In: Carter SK, DiMarco A, Ghione M, Krakoff IH, Mathe G (eds) International symposium on adriamycin. Springer, Berlin Heidelberg New York, p 180

134. Pavone-Macaluso M, Gebbia N, Biondo F, Bertitolini S, Caramia G, Rizzo FP (1976) Permeability of the bladder mucosa to thiotepa, adriamycin, and daunomycin in men and rabbits. Urol Res 4:9

135. Pavone-Macaluso M (1978) Intravesical treatment of superficial (T1) urinary bladder tumors: a review of a 15-year experience. In: WHO, Diagnostics and treatment of superficial urinary bladder tumors. Collaborating centre for research and treatment of urinary bladder cancer, Stockholm, pp 21–36

136. Pavone-Macaluso M, Ingaugiola GB (1980) Local chemotherapy in bladder cancer treatment. Oncology [Suppl] 37:71–76

137. Peck GL, Yoder FW (1976) Treatment of lamellar ichthyosis and other keritinising dermatosis with an oral synthetic retinoid. Lancet 2:1172–1173

138. Poole-Wilson DS, Barnard RJ (1971) Total cystectomy for bladder tumors. Br J Urol 43:16

139. Presant CA, Bearman R, Bartolucci A, Lefant J (1981) Randomized study of 13-cis-retinoic acid (RA) plus busulfan (B) or B alone in chronic phase chronic granulocytic leukemia. Proc Am Soc Clin Oncol 22:488i Abstract

140. Prout GR, Cox E, Cummings KB, Flanagan MJ, Friedell GH, Hodges CV, Koontz WW, Merrin CEA, Schmidt JD, Veenema RJ, Warram JH (1977) Surveillance, initial assessment and subsequent progress of patients with superficial bladder cancer in a prospective longitudinal study. Cancer Res 37:2907

141. Prout GR (1977) Bladder carcinoma and a TNM system of classification. J Urol 117:583
142. Prout GR, Griffin PP, Nocks BN (1981) Intravesical therapy of low stage bladder carcinoma with mitomycin-C: comparison of results in untreated and previously treated patients. Am Urol Assn Proc Abstract 437
143. Pyrah LN, Raper FP, Thomas GM (1964) Report of a follow-up of papillary tumors of the bladder. Br J Urol 36:14
144. Riddle PR (1978) Pre-organized intervention concerning Epodyl treatment. Proceedings of the second course on urologic oncology, E Hore Majorana, Erice Trapani
145. Riddle PR, Wallace DM (1971) Intracavitary chemotherapy for multiple non-invasive bladder tumors. Br J Urol 43:181−184
146. Riddle PR (1973) The management of superficial bladder tumors with intravesical epodyl. Br J Urol 45:84−87
147. Riddle PR, Chisholm GD, Trott PA, Pugh RCB (1976) Flat carcinoma in situ of bladder. Br J Urol 47:829−833
148. Robinson MRG, Shetty MB, Richards B, Bastable J, Glashan RW, Smith PH (1977) Intravesical epodyl in the management of bladder tumors: combined experience of the Yorkshire Urologic Cancer Research Group. J Urol 118:972−973
149. Rozencweig M, Von Hoff DD, Henneny JE, Muggia FM (1977) VM-26 and VP-16-213: a comparative analysis. Cancer 40:334−342
150. Rubben H, Dahm HH, Lutzeyer W (1981) Frequency of recurrences and tumor progression of superficial bladder carcinomas. Urologe [A] 20:211−214
151. Russell M (1963) Treatment of papillary tumor of bladder with chloropactin XCB (oxochlorosene): a preliminary report. J Urol 89:188
152. Sadoughi N, Johnson RA, Ezdinli EZ, Bush IM, Guinan P (1973) Intravesical bleomycin in treatment of carcinoma of the bladder. J Am Med Assoc 226:465
153. Schade ROK, Swinney J (1973) The association of urothelial atypism with neoplasia: its importance in treatment and prognosis. J Urol 109:619
154. Schellhammer PF, Bean MA, Whitmore WF (1977) Prostatic involvement by transitional cell carcinoma: pathogenesis, patterns, and prognosis. J Urol 118:399
155. Schulman CC, Denis LJ, Oosterlinck W, DeSy W, Chantrie M, VanCangh PJ (1981) Early adjuvant adriamycin in superficial bladder cancer. Am Urol Assn Meeting, Abstract 436
156. Schulman C, Sylvester R, Robinson M, Smith P, Lachand A, Denis L, Pavone-Macaluso M, De Pavio M, Staquet M (1982) Adjuvant therapy of T1 bladder carcinoma: preliminary results in an EORTC randomized study. Urol Res (in press)
157. Semple JE (1948) Papillomata of the bladder treated with podophyllin. Br Med J 1:1235
158. Seemayer TA, Knáack J, Thelmo WC (1975) Further observations on carcinoma in situ of the urinary bladder: silent but extensive intraprostatic involvement. Cancer 36:514
159. Smith IM, Lane V, O'Flynn JD (1978) Epodyl in management of noninvasive vesical neoplasms. Urology 11:474−477
160. Smith PH, McCollum CN (1976) Intravesical bleomycin in bladder cancer. J Am Med Assoc 235:906−907
161. Soloway MS (1977) Intravesical and systemic chemotherapy of murine bladder cancer. Cancer Res 37:2918−2929
162. Soloway MS, Murphy W, Rao MK (1978) Serial multiple site biopsies in patients with bladder cancer. J Urol 120:57
163. Soloway MS (1980) Rationale for intensive intravesical chemotherapy for superficial bladder cancer. J Urol 123:461−466
164. Soloway MS, Murphy WM, DeFuria MD (1981) Intravesical mitomycin-C in superficial bladder cancer. Am Soc Clin Oncol Proc 22:469
165. Soto EA, Friedell GH, Tiltman AJ (1977) Bladder cancer as seen in giant histologic sections. Cancer 39:447

166. Sporn MB, Kunlop NM, Newton DL, Smith JM (1976) Prevention of chemical carcinogenesis by Vitamin A and its synthetic analogs (retinoids). Fed Proc 35: 1332–1338
167. Sporn MB, Squire RA, Brown CC, Smith JM, Wenk ML, Springer S (1977) 13-cis-retinoic acid: inhibition of bladder carcinogenesis in the rat. Science 195: 487–489
168. Squire RA, Sporn MB, Brown CC, Smith JM, Wenk ML, Springer S (1977) Histopathological evaluation of the inhibition of rat bladder carcinogenesis by 13-cis-retinoic acid. Cancer Res 37: 2930–2936
169. Swartz D, Flamant R, Lellouch J, Denoix PF (1961) Results of a French survey on the role of tobacco, particularly inhalation, in different cancer sites. J Natl Cancer Inst 26: 1085
170. Thompson N (1960) Bladder papilloma: an analysis of 75 cases. Br J Surg 47: 419–424
171. Turner AG, Hendry WF, Williams GB, Bloom HJG (1977) The treatment of advanced bladder cancer with methotrexate. Br J Urol 49: 673–678
172. Union Internationale Contre le Cancer (1974) TNM classification of malignant tumors. de Buren, Geneva
173. Utz DC, Hanash KA, Farrow GM (1970) The plight of the patient with carcinoma in situ of the bladder. J Urol 103: 160
174. Utz DC, Farrow GM, Rife CC, Segura JW, Zincke H (1980) Carcinoma in situ of the bladder. Cancer 45: 1842–1848
175. Uyama T, Moriwaki S, Nakamura S, Kagawa S (1980) Intravesical instillation of adriamycin combined with low-dose irradiation for superficial bladder cancer. Urology 15: 584–587
176. Van der Werf-Messing B (1978) Cancer of the urinary bladder treated by interstitial radium implant. Int J Radiat Oncol Biol Phys 4: 373–378
177. Van der Werf-Messing B (1969) Carcinoma of the bladder treated by suprapubic radium implants. Eur J Cancer 5: 277–285
178. Van der Werf-Messing B, Hop WCJ (1981) Carcinoma of the urinary bladder (category T1 Nx Mo) treated either by radium implant or by transurethral resection only. Int J Radiat Oncol Biol Phys 7: 299–303
179. Varhavakis MJ, Gaeta J, Moore RH, Murphy GP (1974) Superficial bladder tumor, aspects of clinical progression. Urology 4: 414
180. Veenema RJ, Dean AL, Roberts M, Fingerhut B, Chowhury BK, Tarassoly H (1962) Bladder carcinoma treated by direct instillation of thiotepa. J Urol 88: 60–63
181. Veenema RJ, Dean AL, Uson AC, Roberts M, Longo F (1969) Thiotepa bladder instillations: therapy and prophylaxis for superficial bladder tumors. J Urol 101: 711–715
182. Wallace AC, Herschfield ES (1958) The experimental implantation of tumor cells in the urinary tract. Br J Cancer 12: 622
183. Wallace DM (1971) Intracavitary radiation for multiple non-infiltrating bladder tumors. Br J Urol 43: 177–180
184. Wallace DM, Hindmarsh JR, Webb JN, Busuttil A, Hargreave TB, Newsam JE, Chisholm GD (1979) The role of multiple mucosal biopsies in the management of patients with bladder cancer. Br J Urol 51: 535–540
185. Weldon TE, Soloway MS (1975) Susceptibility of urothelium to neoplastic cellular implantation. Urology 5: 824
186. Westcott JW (1966) The prophylactic use of thiotepa in transitional cell carcinoma of the bladder. J Urol 96: 913–918
187. Whitmore WF (1979) Surgical management of low stage bladder cancer. Semin Oncol 61: 207–216
188. Williams JC, Hammonds JC, Saunders N (1977) T1 bladder tumors. Br J Urol 49: 663
189. Winters WD, Lamm DL (1981) Antibody response to bacillus Calmette-Guerin during immunotherapy in bladder cancer patients. Cancer Res 41: 2672–2676
190. Yagoda A (1980) Chemotherapy of metastatic bladder cancer. Cancer 45: 1879–1888
191. Yoshida O, Brown RR, Bryan GT (1970) Relationship between tryptophan metabolism and heterotopic recurrences of human urinary bladder tumors. Cancer 25: 773

The Chemotherapy of Bladder Carcinoma: Systemic Therapy

W. G. Harker and F. M. Torti

Division of Medical Oncology, Department of Medicine,
Stanford University Medical Center, Stanford, CA 94305, USA

Introduction

While chemotherapy advances in other genitourinary malignancies (e.g., Wilm's tumor and testicular carcinoma) have led to improved disease-free survival and presumed cure, drug therapy of bladder carcinoma remains in a developmental stage. Carcinoma of the urinary bladder ranks seventh in males and 13th in females among causes of death in the United States due to cancer. Approximately 30,000 new cases are reported annually in the U.S. with approximately 10,000 deaths per year attributed to bladder carcinoma [56]. The incidence in males is threefold that in females. Over 60% of these patients are between the ages of 50 and 70 years old [15]. Surgery and radiation are curative modalities. Preoperative staging of the extent of tumor infiltration of the bladder wall is highly predictive of complete resectability and thus probability of cure. While combined modality therapy with preoperative radiotherapy and radical cystectomy has been shown to reduce the loco-regional recurrence rate, there is little evidence that therapy alters the subsequent development of distant metastases [72]. It is not surprising then that the 5-year survival of patients with invasive bladder carcinoma treated with the most expert radiation therapy and surgery, alone or in combination, is between 20% and 50% [16]. Systemic chemotherapy is the only treatment modality with the potential for cure in patients presenting with locally unresectable disease or who develop local or disseminated metastatic involvement after presumed curative initial therapy.

Early chemotherapy trials in patients with bladder carcinoma were less than optimal because of:

1) Selection problems inherent in trials where potentially toxic chemotherapy has to be administered to an elderly patient population with little hope for benefit and considerable opportunity of worsening underlying illness (e.g., underlying heart disease and hypertension).
2) Lack of imaging techniques which would enable one to accurately stage the sites of frequent bladder carcinoma metastases—pelvis, retroperitoneal lymph nodes, and liver—noninvasively. Similarly, accurate measurement of response to therapy for disease in those areas has been impossible.
3) Inadequate use of prospective randomized studies which compare treated patients with an untreated control population.
4) Heterogeneous prior therapy in patients accrued to the chemotherapy trials, i.e., some patients had been treated with surgery alone, some with both surgery and radiation, and some previously given other chemotherapy.
5) Lack of standardization in the reporting of responses.

Recent Results in Cancer Research. Vol. 85
© Springer-Verlag Berlin · Heidelberg 1983

More encouraging is the fact that recent radiologic advances (computerized axial tomography and ultrasonography) are now routinely available at larger centers and allow for more accurate assessment of tumor response. Furthermore, several new chemotherapeutic agents have been shown to have activity against bladder carcinoma in phase I and II trials. Standard criterion for response—complete response (CR), partial response (PR), and nonresponse (NR) or progression (Prog) — have also been better defined. What remains to be demonstrated are the doses, schedules and possible combinations of the active agents that will yield the highest response rates with the least morbidity.

Single Agents

Alkylators

Although available for use since the 1960s this group of non-cell-cycle-specific agents has been inadequately evaluated. As early as 1965, Fox [20] reported that four of eight patients given intravenous cyclophosphamide for bladder carcinoma responded (two objective and two subjective responses). The duration of response was very short (3—6 weeks) but the doses and schedule of administration were quite different from the current intermittent high-dose schedule now felt to be optimal for cyclophosphamide. De Kernion [16] noted responses in four of his ten patients with metastatic disease while Merrin et al. [37] using doses of 1 g/m^2 every 3 weeks obtained responses in 11 of 21 patients (52%). Only four of Merrin's patients had advanced stage D disease, however, one of the four had objective tumor regression. In Yagoda's review of alkylator therapy in 1980 [77], 98 bladder carcinoma patients had been treated with cyclophosphamide with an overall response rate of 31%. Using current strict criterion for response, Yagoda et al. [79] were able to find only two partial responses in 26 cyclophosphamide-treated patients. Certainly, further trials utilizing cyclophospham-ide are warranted. Studies with the remainder of the alkylators — chlorambucil, melphalan, nitrogen mustard, and the nitrosoureas — have not been reported.

Antimetabolites

5-Fluorouracil. This inhibitor of thymidylate synthetase has been available, like cyclophosphamide, for clinical trials since the early 1960s. Unfortunately, the reports of most of the earliest trials do not cover the stage, disease sites, or definition of response. Response rates thus range from 0%—75% in these trials. Glenn et al. [23] in 1963 reported on nine patients with stage $O-D_2$ disease who were treated either with 5-fluorouracil (5-FU) alone, 5-FU plus radiation therapy, or 5-FU used as an adjuvant to surgery. No responses were seen in five patients with "extensively and deeply invasive carcinoma of the bladder", whereas four patients with superficial tumors had favorable objective and subjective responses. Moore et al. [40] noted one CR and five PRs in nine patients treated as part of a broad phase II drug-oriented study. Sites of tumor involvement in these patients are not available. De Kernion [16] and Weiss et al. [70] reported no responses in separate series of six patients each. In contrast, Wilson [75] demonstrated ten responses (one slight and nine good) in a total of 12 patients. Prout et al. [50], in the only prospective randomized trial utilizing 5-FU to date, compared 5-FU to placebo in a small group of patients. Unfortunately, the number of patients with metastatic tumor was small but no significant activity of the 5-FU over placebo could be demonstrated. Though 5-FU has been used in combination trials and probably does have modest antitumor activity against bladder carcinoma, the exact level of that activity is not clear from the literature.

Methotrexate. Folic acid antagonists were first used in the treatment of bladder carcinomas by Sullivan [62], who administered the drug intraarterially and noted "a sustained clinical benefit and decrease in tumor size". Subsequent reports by Andrews and Wilson [4], Burfield [8], Pavone-Macaluso [47], and Altman et al. [1] suggested that methotrexate would be a valuable agent, but the patient numbers were small. In a review and compilation of methotrexate trials up to 1974, Hall et al. [25] found an overall response rate of 36% (10 of 28). In the same review, Hall reported on a series of 42 patients treated at the Royal Marsden Hospital in London with various tumor stages and prior treatment. Their patients were given methotrexate every 1–2 weeks in doses of 50–100 mg IV along with oral furosemide. Of the 42 patients, 11 (26%) showed evidence of tumor regression for periods of 2–20 months. In an update and extension of that series from the Royal Marsden Hospital, Turner et al. [66] reported on 61 patients with bladder carcinoma treated with one of three regimens: a) 50 mg IV, b) 100 mg IV, and c) 200 mg IM with folinic acid rescue, given every 2 weeks. The overall response rates in the three groups were 13% (0/23 CR, 3/23 PR), 56% (3/22 CR, 9/22 PR), and 50% (1/16 CR, 7/16 PR), respectively. One patient achieved a complete remission with disappearance of pulmonary lesions for over 20 months. Finally, Natale et al. [41] reported on a group of 49 patients with urothelial tumors treated as part of a drug-oriented phase II trial with methotrexate given in doses of either 0.5–1.0 mg/kg IV weekly (40 patients) or 250 mg/m^2 via 2 h IV infusion with leucovorin rescue every 2–3 weeks (nine patients). Of 42 evaluable patients, 11 had responses (26%). Partial responses was seen in one of nine patients given the high-dose methotrexate versus 10 of 33 given the lower doses. The response rate in previously untreated patients was higher (38%–6 of 16) than in patients previously treated with chemotherapy (19%).
Methotrexate has demonstrated activity against transitional cell carcinoma of the bladder and warrants inclusion in future combination chemotherapy trials. It would appear from this preliminary report by Natale that low-dose weekly methotrexate is at least as effective, if not more so, than the high-dose regimen.

Antibiotics

Doxorubicin. (Adriamycin). Doxorubicin has been extensively studied in patients with transitional cell carcinoma of the urinary bladder. The combined experience of four groups [7, 38, 43, 68] was reviewed by Carter and Wasserman in 1975 [10] with 30 responses demonstrated in 87 evaluable patients (35% response rate). In a subsequent small series, Weinstein and Schmidt [69] treated 23 patients with stage C-D$_2$ carcinoma of the bladder with doxorubicin every 3 weeks. Though 10 of the 19 evaluable patients had subjective responses (pain relief, etc.) only one patient (5%) was shown to have partial regression of the tumor. Yagoda [80] used five different doxorubicin doses and schedules in treating 35 patients. Only five (14%) "clinically useful responses" were found (1 CR, 4 PRs). Regression was found usually within 3–4 weeks and lasted

1–5 months. Of particular interest is the observation that one patient who failed a trial of doxorubicin at 45 mg/m^2 later responded to a dose of 75 mg/m^2 suggesting that higher doses (60–75 mg/m^2) might be more beneficial.

When stricter criteria for response are applied in doxorubicin trials it appears that the response rate for doxorubicin falls from the initial 35% to the 5%–20% range [22, 69, 80]. If Yagoda's observation regarding higher doses being more effective is correct then special approaches will be necessary to avoid the dose-limiting cardiac toxicity (congestive heart failure and arrythmias-frequent sequellae of cumulative doses over 450–550 mg/m^2) in patients responsive to the drug. It is especially important to this group of patients since over 60% are above the age of 50 years old and are at added risk of suffering from the cardiac toxicity [68]. Current techniques under investigation which might prevent the toxicity include low-dose weekly administration [11, 71] and long-term continuous infusion [32]. Hopefully, these modifications will allow the continued use of doxorubicin both singly and in drug combinations in responding patients who would otherwise have to stop treatment at an arbitrary dose of 450–550 mg/m^2.

Mitomycin C. With demonstrated activity against superficial bladder tumors when given intravesically [47], this antibiotic antitumor agent has seen limited use in metastatic bladder carcinoma because of dose-limiting delayed myelosuppression. Pavone-Macaluso [47] reported seven 'fair' and four 'good' responses in 23 treated patients. Objective remissions were seen in 4 of 19 patients (21%) given mitomycin C at doses of 0.25–0.5 mg/kg IV every 2 weeks by Early et al. [17]. Omura et al. [44] have reported that mitomycin C induced tumor regression in two of their six patients with urinary bladder tumors.

The use of parenteral mitomycin C in combination with other drugs would seem warranted given the overall response rate of 20% in patients treated with mitomycin as a single agent. When given in a schedule every 6 weeks in combination with doxorubicin and 5-FU (which are given every 3 weeks) for gastric carcinoma, mitomycin C produced only moderate bone marrow suppression despite the addition of two other myelosuppressive agents [33].

Cis-diamminedichloroplatinum II

The most active agent in bladder cancer to date, cis-diamminedichloroplatinum (cisplatin) has demonstrated activity in several genitourinary tumors including prostate, testicular, and ovarian carcinomas. Initial response rates of 33% were reported by Yagoda [78] using cisplatin doses of 1.6 mg/kg IV every 3 weeks in early trials and 70 mg/m^2 every 3 weeks in later trials. The response rate approached 50% (10 of 21) in previously untreated patients. Soloway [58] and Rosoff et al. [52] using similar doses and schedules noted responses in 47% and 33% of their patients, respectively. Merrin [36] reported an overall response rate of 37.2% in 51 patients with one complete clinical response lasting 5 months and 18 PRs also lasting an average of 5 months. More recently, Herr [26] obtained 3 CRs and 6 PRs in 21 previously untreated patients using cisplatin as a single agent. The duration of the CRs was greater than 12 months. Soloway et al. [60] in an update of his original series report no CRs, however, and nine PRs in a group of 27 patients treated with 70 mg/m^2 given every 3 weeks. An additional 12 patients had stabilization of their disease. While there was a survival benefit for patients achieving a PR or disease stability versus the nonresponders (78%, 84%, and 17% probability of surviving 6 months, respectively), no survival difference was found between partial responders and those with disease stabilization.

Initially, the nephrotoxicity of cisplatin limited its use in clinical trials but with studies showing that appropriate hydration and diuresis as well as changes in infusion duration [29] can markedly reduce the incidence of tubular damage, this drug has gained acceptance in many tumor types. The use of newer antiemetics such as metoclopramide [24] will hopefully eliminate or control the severe nausea and vomiting which accompanies the administration of this effective agent. The onset of response in cisplatin-treated patients is usually between 7 and 14 days with objective tumor regression usually occurring within 4−6 weeks [78]. While a few long-term responders have been reported, the usual duration of response is 5−6 months. New platinum analogs, which do not induce renal abnormalities and are less emetigenic, are in the developmental stages and should allow for longer term administration in responding patients.

Vinca Alkaloids

Prior investigation of the activity of these mitotic-spindle inhibitors (vinblastine and vincristine) in urothelial tumors has been limited to phase I and II studies in heavily pretreated patients. Holland et al. [27] in one such study reported three responses in ten patients with bladder carcinoma treated with 25−75 µg/kg vincristine weekly. Pavone-Macaluso [47] obtained one 'good' response in seven patients treated with vinblastine alone. Blumenreich et al. [6] noted PRs in 5 of 28 (18%) patients treated with vinblastine at doses of 0.10−0.15 mg/kg weekly. The PRs lasted 2−5 months. Two of the nine responses were in previously untreated patients while of the 19 patients who had received prior chemotherapy three responded. Since some degree of antitumor activity was found in these preliminary studies, further trials are necessary to define the activity of both vinblastine and vincristine as single agents and combined with other active drugs.

Miscellaneous Agents

Several other agents with activity in other tumor types have either not been tested against bladder carcinoma or have had too little use to allow comment on their activity. These drugs include the podophyllotoxin derivatives VM-26 and VP-16-213, Neocarsinostatin, hexamethylmelamine, bleomycin, as well as the nitrosoureas. Several of these drugs are listed in Table 1. Another area needing further exploration is the question of what activity the new biologic response modifiers (e.g., interferon [28] and thymosin) will demonstrate against this tumor type. Further disease-oriented phase II trials at institutions treating larger numbers of patients with bladder cancer or as part of cooperative group trials will be necessary to define the activity of these drugs. The use of the FANFT tumor model [59] and in vitro techniques for cloning human tumor cells hold promise as ways of screening newer agents for human trials.

Table 1. Single agent activity in advanced bladder carcinoma

Drug	Number of patients	Average % response	Reference
Bleomycin (Bilharzal)	58	9	[21]
Cyclophosphamide	98	31	[16, 20, 37, 77]
Doxorubicin	235+	23	[10, 16, 63]
5-Fluorouracil	75+	35	[10]
Hexamethylmelamine	36	36	[5, 76]
Methotrexate	140	29	[1, 4, 8, 41, 47, 66]
Mitomycin C	48	21	[17, 44, 47]
Neocarsinostatin	18	6	[42]
	17	70	[54]
Cis-Platinum	188	33	[18, 36, 49, 53, 58, 60, 78]
PALA	12	0	[77]
VP-16-213	21	5	[45, 77]
VM-26	29	20	[35, 48, 77]
Vinblastine	35	17	[6, 47]
Vincristine	11	27	[27, 47]
Yoshi 864	11	18	[2]

Combination Regimens

Since single agent responses tend to be limited in number and durability, attempts have been made to improve on the quantity and quality of responses by using two or more active drugs in combination. The various combinations have been chosen either empirically or on the basis of sequencing data obtained in the murine bladder cancer model [59]. While theoretically the use of several drugs will lessen the possibility of intrinsic biochemical resistance in carcinoma cells, other factors of probable equal importance such as low growth fraction and regional tumor hypoxia and hypoperfusion are not affected. Biochemical resistance can be combated by the development of new drugs. In addition, cytokinetic factors, such as sequential drug scheduling and hypoxic cell sensitizers, are currently being evaluated.

Cisplatin, with the highest activity of any single agent to date against bladder carcinoma, has been used as the nucleus for a considerable number of combination chemotherapy trials. The discussion of the various combinations will be divided into cisplatin-containing regimens and those without cisplatin.

Cisplatin-containing Regimens

Cisplatin has been used in combination with cyclophosphamide, doxorubicin, cyclophosphamide and doxorubicin, and 5-FU plus doxorubicin (see Table 2). The majority of these trials contain small patient numbers and lack appropriate control groups treated with cisplatin only. Yagoda [77, 78] observed responses in 54% of 26 patients given 70 mg/m^2 cisplatin, and $45-60 \text{ mg/m}^2$ doxorubicin; 43% in 35 patients treated with 70 mg/m^2 cisplatin, and $250-1000 \text{ mg/m}^2$ cyclophosphamide; and 50% in 28 patients who had received 70 mg/m^2 cisplatin on day 1, 250 mg/m^2 cyclophosphamide on day 2, and $30-45 \text{ mg/m}^2$ doxorubicin on day 3. Responses in

Table 2. Cis-platinum-containing combination regimens for advanced bladder carcinoma

Drugs	No. of patients	No. responding	% response	Reference
Cis-platinum + cyclophosphamide	32	15	47	[78]
Cis-platinum + cyclophosphamide	47	6	12.7	[18]
Cis-platinum + doxorubicin	26	14	54	[78]
Cis-platinum + doxorubicin	36	13	36	[22]
Cis-platinum + doxorubicin	1	0	0	[67]
Cis-platinum + doxorubicin	1	0	0	[39]
Cis-platinum + cyclophosphamide + doxorubicin	50	26	52	[55]
Cis-platinum + cyclophosphamide + doxorubicin	23	19	83	[30]
Cis-platinum + cyclophosphamide + doxorubicin	15	2	13	[9]
Cis-platinum + cyclophosphamide + doxorubicin	12	10	90	[61]
Cis-platinum + cyclophosphamide + doxorubicin	9	4	44	[65]
Cis-platinum + cyclophosphamide + doxorubicin	6	3	50	[78]
Cis-platinum + doxorubicin + 5-fluorouracil	16	10	62.5	[74]
Cis-platinum + doxorubicin + 5-fluorouracil	39	18	46.2	[73]

previously untreated patients (67%) were higher than in patients previously treated with chemotherapy (50%). Vogl et al. [67], Mills et al. [39], and Gagliano [22] all found fewer responding patients than did Yagoda with the combination of cisplatin and doxorubicin (0/1, 0/1, and 13/36 patients, respectively). Gagliano reported, however, that the cisplatin and doxorubicin combination was more effective than cisplatin alone (8 of 40 responded – 20%). While the difference between the overall response rates in the two groups did not reach statistical significance, the median survival of responders (42 weeks) was significantly better than those with stable disease (26 weeks) or progression (15 weeks). Einstein et al. [18] in reporting results of a National Bladder Cancer Collaborative Group A study found only six PRs in 47 previously untreated patients given cisplatin and doxorubicin.

In a very encouraging preliminary report of a pilot study, Sternberg et al. [61] achieved a remarkable 83% response rate (10 of 12 patients) using 100 mg/m^2 cisplatin on day 2, 50 mg/m^2 doxorubicin on day 1, and 650 mg/m^2 cyclophosphamide on day 1 (CISCA). Responses were seen in six of seven patients with lung involvement and two of three with bony disease. When recently updated and expanded, the series now of 41 patients has 17 responders (42%) [55]. The Eastern Cooperative Oncology Group (ECOG) [31] has randomized 98 patients to treatment with either the three-drug regimen – cisplatin, doxorubicin, and cyclophosphamide – or cisplatin alone. Though the randomization assignments of the study remain coded the overall response rates are not significantly different – 24% vs 34%, respectively. Three smaller nonrandomized trials have produced marked disparate results with responses of 82% (19/23) [30], 44%

(4/9) [65], and 13% (2/15) [9] using similar doses of cisplatin, doxorubicin, and cyclophosphamide as described above. Clearly, prospective randomized trials are needed comparing the two- and three-drug combinations with cisplatin alone. Finally, Williams et al. [74] drawing from preliminary experience with doxorubicin and 5-FU combinations (see below) were able to obtain a 62.5% response rate in 16 patients given cisplatin, doxorubicin, and 5-FU every 3 weeks. The update of the study in 1979, however, revealed that the rate of response had fallen to 46.2% (18/39) [73]. Of note is the fact that these drugs produced no CRs; there did not appear to be a survival advantage from achieving a response; and the responses tended to be of short duration (4−6 months).

The results of the cisplatin combination chemotherapy trials in bladder carcinoma fail to demonstrate clear superiority of the combinations when compared with cisplatin use alone.

Combinations Not Containing Cisplatin

The non-cisplatin containing regimens can be seen in Table 3. Attention is drawn to the wide range of responses obtained by different investigators with apparently similar regimens. Also of note is the paucity of controlled trials comparing the two- or three-drug combinations with single agent chemotherapy alone. Certainly, the responses reported with cisplatin alone compare favorably with the 40%−50% responses seen in the larger series noted here. The advantages of these regimens relate to the fact that they do not contain cisplatin with its associated gastrointestinal and renal toxicity. Most of them do contain doxorubicin, however, making the previously described cardiotoxicity a limiting factor in proper drug combination selection.

Table 3. Combination regimens for advanced bladder carcinoma (non-platinum containing)

Drugs	No. of patients	No. responding	% response	Reference
Doxorubicin + cyclophosphamide	18	9	50	[37]
Doxorubicin + cyclophosphamide	17	3	17	[79]
Doxorubicin + 5-fluorouracil	85	35	41	[14, 19, 34]
Doxorubicin + VM-26	27	5	19	[51]
Doxorubicin + cyclophosphamide + 5-fluorouracil	21	3	14	[57]
Doxorubicin + cyclophosphamide + 5-fluorouracil	3	2	66	[12, 13]
Doxorubicin + cyclophosphamide + methotrexate	26	10	38	[64]
5-fluorouracil + vinblastine	4	2	50	[3]
Cyclophosphamide + 5-fluorouracil + methotrexate + vincristine + Ca + actinomycin D	4	2	50	[49]
Cyclophosphamide + hydroxyurea + vinblastine + vincristine	18	4	22	[46]

Conclusions

Three drugs have activity against transitional cell carcinoma of the urinary bladder — cisplatin, doxorubicin, and methotrexate. Three other agents probably are active but to a lesser degree — cyclophosphamide, mitomycin C and 5-fluorouracil. Further study is necessary to define the activity of the latter three drugs as well as bleomycin, VM-26, VP-16-213, the vinca alkaloids, hexamethylmelamine, and the nitrosoureas. Cisplatin appears to be the most active chemotherapeutic agent but the duration of responses is short (less than 6 months) when this drug is used alone. There does not appear to be a clear demonstration of superiority of any of the cisplatin combination regimens over that of cisplatin alone with regard to response rate, duration of response, or overall survival.

Recent advances in ultrasonography and computerized axial tomography allow for the accurate assessment of disease status prior to treatment and measurement of tumor responsiveness in areas like the pelvis and retroperitoneum, which were previously inaccessible without surgery.

Since only 20%–50% of bladder carcinoma patients with stages B_2–D will survive 5 years despite optimal surgical and radiotherapy techniques [16], consideration should be given to adjuvant trials using single agent cisplatin alone or in combination with doxorubicin and cyclophosphamide for optimally resected patients with high risk of recurrence. Once recurrence has been documented, consideration should be given to placement of patients with measurable disease on phase II studies to expedite the evaluation of the newer chemotherapeutic agents and/or biologic response modifiers.

References

1. Altman CC, McCague NJ, Ripepi AC, Cardoza M (1972) The use of methotrexate in advanced carcinoma of the bladder. J Urol 198: 217–273
2. Altman S: Yoshi 864 (1978) 1 propanol, 3,3'-Iminodi-dimethane sulfonate (ester) hydrochloride: A phase II study in solid tumors. Cancer Treat Rep 62: 389–395
3. Al-Sarraf M, Amer MH, Vaitkevicius VK (1977) Chemotherapy and survival in patients with urinary bladder cancer. Proc AACR and ASCO 18: 146
4. Andrews MC, Wilson WL (1976) Phase II study of methotrexate (NSC-740) in solid tumors. Cancer Chemother Rep 51: 471–474
5. Blum RH, Livingston RB, Carter SK (1973) Hexamethylmelamine — a new drug with activity in solid tumors. Eur J Cancer 9: 195–202
6. Blumenreich M, Yagoda A, Watson RC, Needles B (1981) Phase II trial of vinblastine sulfate (VLB) in transitional cell carcinoma. Proc ASCO 22: 466
7. Bonadonna G, Monfardini S, DeLena M, Fossati-Bellani F, Beretta G (1972) Clinical Trials with Adriamycin — results of three year study. In: Carter SK, DiMarco A, Ghione M (eds) International symposium on adriamycin. Springer New York, 139–152
8. Burfield GD (1972) Intravenous methotrexate in the treatment of advanced bladder cancer. Br J Urol 44: 121–124
9. Campbell M, Baker LH, Opipaui M, Al-Sarraf M (1981) Phase II trial with cisplatin, doxorubicin, cyclophosphamide (CAP) in the treatment of urothelial cell carcinoma. Cancer Treat Rep 65: 897–899
10. Carter SK, Wasserman TH (1975) The chemotherapy of urologic cancer. Cancer 36: 729–747

11. Chlebowski RT, Paroly WS, Pugh RP, Hueser J, Jacobs EM, Pajak TF, Bateman JR (1980) Adriamycin given as a weekly schedule without a loading course: clinical effective with reduced incidence of cardiotoxicity. Cancer Treat Rep 64: 47–51
12. Collier D, Soloway MS (1976) Doxorubicin hydrochloride, cyclophosphamide, a 5-fluorouracil combination in advanced prostate and transitional cell carcinoma. Urology 8: 459–464
13. Corder MP, Cicmil GA (1976) Effective treatment of metastatic squamous cell carcinoma of the prostate with adriamycin. J Urol 155: 222
14. Cross RJ, Glashan RW, Humphrey CS, Robinson MRG, Smith PH, Williams RE (1976) Treatment of advanced bladder cancer with adriamycin and 5-fluorouracil. Br J Urol 48: 609–615
15. Dean AL, Mostofi FK, Thomson RU, Clark RL (1954) A restudy of the first 1400 tumors in the bladder tumor registry, AFIP. J Urol 71: 571–590
16. de Kernion JB (1977) The chemotherapy of advanced bladder carcinoma. Cancer Res 37: 2771–2774
17. Early K, Elias EG, Mittelson A, Albert D, Murph GP (1973) Mitomycin C in the treatment of metastatic transitional cell carcinoma of the bladder. Cancer 31: 1150–1153
18. Einstein A, Soloman M, Corder M, Bonney W, Coombs J (1981) Diamine dichloroplatinum (DDP) vs DDP plus cyclophosphamide (CY) for metastatic bladder carcinoma. A National Bladder Cancer Collaborative Group A (NBCCGA) study. Proc ASCO 22: 461
19. EORTC (1977) The treatment of advanced carcinoma of the bladder with a combination of adriamycin and 5-FU. Eur Urol 3: 276–278
20. Fox M (1965) The effect of cyclophosphamide on some urinary tract tumors. Br J Urol 37: 399–403
21. Gad-El-Mawla NM, Ziegler JL (1978) Phase II trial of bleomycin in bilharzal bladder cancer. Cancer Treat Rep 62: 1109–1110
22. Gagliano R (1980) Adriamycin versus adriamycin plus cisplatin in transitional cell bladder carcinoma. A SWOG study. Proc ASCO 21: 347
23. Glenn J, Hunt L, Cathem J (1963) Chemotherapy of bladder cancer with 5-Fluorouracil. Cancer Chemother Rep 27: 67–69
24. Gralla RJ, Itri LM, Pisko SE, Squillante AE, Kelsen DP, Braun DW, Jr, Bordin LA, Braun TJ, Young CW (1982) Antiemetic efficacy of high-dose metoclophramide: randomized trails with placebo and prochlorperazine in patients with chemotherapy-induced nausea and vomiting. N Engl J Med 305: 905–909
25. Hall RR, Bloom HJG, Freeman JE, Nawrocki A, Wallace DM (1971) Methotrexate treatment for advanced bladder cancer. Br J Urol 46: 431–438
26. Herr HW (1980) Cis-diamminedichloride platinum (II) in the treatment of advanced bladder cancer. J Urol 853–855
27. Holland JF, Scharlan C, Gailani S, Krant MJ, Olson KB, Horton J, Shnider BF, Lynch JJ, Owens A. Carbone PP, Colby J, Grob D, Miller SP, Hall TC (1973) Vincristine treatment of advanced cancer. A cooperative study of 392 cases. Cancer Res 33: 1258–1264
28. Ikic D, Maricic Z, Oresic V, Rode B, Nola P, Smudj K, Knezevic M, Jusic D (1981) Application of human leucocyte interferon in patients with urinary bladder papillomatosis, breast cancer and melanoma. Lancet 1: 1022–1024
29. Jacobs C, Bertino JR, Goffinet DR, Fee WR, Goode RL (1978) 24-hour infusion of cisplatinum in head and neck cancers. Cancer 42: 2135–2140
30. Kedia KR, Gibbons C, Persky L (1981) The management of advanced bladder carcinoma. J Urol 125: 655–658
31. Khandekar JD, Elson PJ, DeWys WD, Slayton R (1981) Comparative activity and toxicity of cis-diammine-dichloroplatinum (DDP) vs cyclophosphamide (CTX) Adriamycin (ADR) and DDP (CAD) in disseminated transitional cell carcinomas of the urinary tract (DTCUT). Proc ASCO 22: 461

32. Legha SS, Benjamin RS, Mackay B, Ewer M, Wallace S, Valdivieso M, Rasmussen SL, Blumenschein GR, Freireich EJ (1982) Reductin of doxorubicin cardiotoxicity by prolonged continous intravenous infusion. Ann Intern Med 46: 133–139
33. Macdonald JS, Schein PS, Wooley PV, Smythe T, Ueno W, Hoth D, Smith F, Boiron M, Gisselbrecht C, Brunet R, Lagarde C (1980) 5-fluorouracil, doxorubicin and mitomycin (FAM) combination chemotherapy for advanced gastric cancer. Ann Int Med 43: 533–536
34. Martino S, Samal B, Al-Sarraf M (1980) Phase II study of 5-fluorouracil and adriamycin in transitional cell carcinoma of the urinary tract. Cancer Treat Rep 64: 161–163
35. Mechl Z, Rovny F, Sopkova B (1977) VM-26 (4 demethyl-epipodo phyllotoxin-B-d-theonylidine glucoside) in the treatment of urinary bladder tumors. Neoplasma 24 (4): 411
36. Merrin C (1975) Treatment of advanced bladder cancer with cisdiammine dichloroplatinum (II) (NSC 119875): a pilot study. J Urol 114: 884–887
37. Merrin C, Cartegena R, Wajsman Z, Baumgardner C, Murphy GP (1975) Chemotherapy of bladder cancer with cytoxan and adriamycin. J Urol 114: 884–887
38. Middleman E, Luce J, Frei E (1971) Clinical trials with adriamycin. Cancer 28: 844–850
39. Mills RC, Maurer LH, Forcier RJ, Grace WR, Burke GP, Karp DO, Smith RL, McIntyre OR, Bean C (1977) Clinical trial of combined therapy with adriamycin and cisdichlorodiammineplatinum (II). Cancer Treat Rep 61: 477–479
40. Moore G, Bross ID, Ausman R, Nadler S, Jones R, Slack N, Reimm A (1963) Effects of 5-fluorouracil (NSC 19893) in 389 patients with cancer. Cancer Chemother Rep 27: 67–69
41. Natale RB, Yagoda A, Watson RC, Whitmore WF, Blumenreich M, Brain DW, Jr (1981) Methotrexate: an active drug in bladder cancer. Cancer 47: 1246–1250
42. Natale RB, Yagoda A, Watson RC, Stover DE (1980) Phase II trial of neocarzinostatin in patients with bladder and prostate cancer: toxicity of a five day I.V. bolus schedule. Cancer 45: 2836–2842
43. O'Bryan RM, Luce JK, Talley TW, Gottlieb JA, Baker LH, Bonadonna G (1973) Phase II evaluation of adriamycin in human neoplasia. Cancer 32: 1–8
44. Omura J, Okita K, Tasaka S (1962) Chemotherapy of cancer of the urinary bladder. Bull Cancer Inst Okayama Univ 2: 143–156
45. Panduro J, Hansen M, Hansen HH (1981) Oral VP-16-213 in transitional cell carcinoma of the bladder: A Phase II study. Cancer Treat Rep 65: 703–704
46. Pannuti F, Martoni A, Casadio M, Fruet F, Belfiore G (1979) New regimen of combination chemotherapy (CHVV) in the treatment of advanced bladder cancer: a pilot study. Cancer Treat Rep 63: 1427–1428
47. Pavone-Macaluso M (1971) Chemotherapy of vesical and prostatic tumors. Br J Urol 43: 701–708
48. Pavone-Macaluso M (1976) EORTC genitourinary tract cooperative group: a single-day chemotherapy of bladder cancer with adriamycin, VM-26, or bleomycin. Eur Urol 2: 138
49. Price LA, Goldie JH (1971) Multiple drug therapy for disseminated malignant tumors. Br Med J 4: 336–339
50. Prout GR, Bross IDJ, Slack NH, Ausman RK (1968) Carcinoma of the bladder, 5-fluorouracil and the critical role of a placebo: a cooperative group report. I. Cancer 22: 926–931
51. Rodriguez LH, Johnson DE, Holoye PY, Samuels MC (1977) Combination VM-26 and adriamycin for metastatic transitional cell carcinoma. Cancer Treat Rep 61: 87–88
52. Rossof AH, Talley RW, Stephens RL (1977) Phase II evaluation of single high dose cisdiammine dichloroplatinum (II) (NCS-119875, CACP) in gynecologic (GYN) and genitourinary (GU) neoplasia. Proc ASCR and ASCO 18: 99

53. Rossof AH, Talley RW, Stephens R, Thigpen T, Samson MK, Groppe C, Eyre HJ, Fisher R (1979) Phase II evaluation of cis dichlorodiammineplatinum (II) in advanced malignancies of the genitourinary and gynecologic organs: a Southwest Oncology Group Study. Cancer Treat Rep 63: 1557–1564

54. Sakamoto S, Ogata J, Ikegami K, Naeda H (1978) Effects of systemic administration of neocarsinostatin, a new protein antibiotic on human bladder cancer. Cancer Treat Rep 62: 453–454

55. Samuels ML, Logothetis C, Trindade A, Johnson PE (1980) Cytoxan, adriamycin and cisplatinum (CISCA) in metastatic bladder cancer. Proc AACR 21: 137

56. Silverberg E (1978) Cancer Statistics, CA 28: 17–30

57. Swalley RV, Bartolucci AA, Hemstret G, Hester M (1981) A phase II evaluation of a 3 drug combination of cyclophosphamide, doxorubicin, and 5-fluorouracil in patients with advanced bladder carcinoma or stage D prostate cancer. J Urol 125: 191–195

58. Soloway MS (1978) Cis diammine dichloroplatinum (II)(DDP) in advanced bladder cancer. Proc ASCO 19: 366

59. Soloway MS (1977) Intravesical and systemic chemotherapy of murine bladder cancer. Cancer Res 37: 2918–2929

60. Soloway MS, Jicard M, Ford K (1981) Cis-diamminedichloroplatinum (II) in locally advanced and metastatic cancer. Cancer 47: 476–480

61. Sternberg JJ, Bracken RB, Handel PB, Johnson DE (1977) Combination chemotherapy (CISCA) for advanced urinary tract carcinoma: a preliminary report. JAMA 238: 2282–2287

62. Sullivan RD (1962) Intra-arterial methotrexate therapy: The dose, duration and route of administration studies of methotrexate in clinical cancer chemotherapy. In: Porter R, Wiltshaw E (eds) First symposium on methotrexate in the treatment of cancer. Wright Bristol 50–55

63. Tan C, Etcubanas E, Wollner N, Rosen G, Gilladoga A, Showel J, Murphy ML, Krakoff IH (1973) Adriamycin – an antitumor antibiotic in treatment of neoplastic disease. Cancer 32: 9–17

64. Tannock I, Gospodarowicz M, Evans WK (1981) Methotrexate, adriamycin and cyclophosphamide (MAC) chemotheraphy for transitional cell carcinoma of the urinary tract. Proc ASCO 461

65. Troner M, Hemstreet G (1978) Cyclophosphamide, adriamycin and cisplatin (CAP) chemotherapy of metastatic transitional cell carcinoma of the bladder. Proc AACR 19: 161

66. Turner AG, Hendry WF, Williams GB, Bloom HJG (1977) The treatment of advanced bladder carcinoma with methotrexate. Br J Urol 49: 673–678

67. Vogl S, Ohnuma T, Perloff M, Holland JF (1976) Combination chemotherapy with adriamycin and cis-diamminedichloroplatinum in patients with metastatic diseases. Cancer 38: 21–26

68. Von Hoff DD, Layard MW, Basa P, Davis HL, Jr., Von Hoff AL, Rozencweig M, Muggia FM (1979) Risk factors for doxorubicin-induced congestive heart failure. Ann Intern Med 91: 710–717

69. Weinstein S, Schmidt J (1976) Doxorubicin chemotherapy in advanced transitional cell carcinoma. Urology 8: 336–341

70. Weiss A, Jackson L, Carabasi R (1961) An evaluation of 5-fluorouracil in malignant disease. Ann Intern Med 55: 731–741

71. Weiss AJ, Manthel RW (1977) Experience with the use of adriamycin in combination with other anticancer agents using a weekly schedule, with particular reference to lack of cardiac toxicity. Cancer 40: 2046–2052

72. Whitmore WF Jr, Batata MA, Ghoneim MA, Grabstald H, Unal A, (1977) Radical cystectomy with or without prior irradiation in the treatment of bladder cancer. J Urol 118: 184–187

73. Williams SD, Einhorn LH, Donohue JP (1979) Cisplatin Combination chemotherapy of bladder cancer. Cancer Clin Trials 2:335–338
74. Williams SD, Rohn RJ, Donohue JP, Einhorn LH (1978) Chemotherapy of bladder cancer with cis-diamminedichloroplatinum (DDP), adriamycin (ADR), and 5-fluorouracil (5-FU). Proc ASCO 19:316
75. Wilson WL (1960) Chemotherapy of human solid tumors with 5-fluorouracil. Cancer 13:1230–1239
76. Wilson WL, Schroeder JN, Bisel HF, Mrazek R, Hummel RP (1969) Phase II study of hexamethylmelamine (NSC 13875). Cancer 23:132–136
77. Yagoda A (1980) Chemotherapy of metastatic bladder cancer. Cancer 45:1879–1888
78. Yagoda A (1979) Phase II trials with cisdiamminedichloride II in the treatment of urothelial cancers. Cancer Treat Rep 63:1565–1572
79. Yagoda A, Watson RC, Grabstald H, Barzell WE, Whitmore WF (1977) Adriamycin and cyclophosphamide in advanced bladder cancer. Cancer Treat Rep 61:97–99
80. Yagoda A, Watson RC, Whitmore WF, Grabstadt H, Middleman MP, Krakoff IH (1977) Adriamycin in advanced urinary tract cancer. Experience in 42 patients and review of the literature. Cancer 39:279–285

Response Criteria in Urologic Malignancies

F. M. Torti

Division of Medical Oncology, Stanford University Medical Center, Palo Alto, CA, USA

Prostate Cancer

The recognition of a response to treatment in prostatic carcinoma is not qualitatively different than that in other solid tumors; nonetheless, the preponderance of bone as a site of metastases in prostate cancer makes effective measurement of response difficult. In other disease sites, such as colorectal cancer or lung cancer, inability to detect early and quantitative changes on bone scan (i.e., 25% versus 50% improvement) are of less clinical importance. In these tumors there are indicator lesions in lung, soft tissue, etc. which can be easily measured and quantitated. In contrast, in prostatic carcinoma, for the vast majority of patients, bone is the only site of metastatic disease and the dominant site of symptomatic disease.

The current inability to quantitate objectively changes in disease over time (in bone, in the prostatic bed, etc.) seriously impairs the investigation of new agents and new approaches to patients with metastatic disease [30]. Prostatic cancer patients have been excluded from drug-oriented phase II trials because bone disease has been considered 'nonmeasurable' disease. Since the disease is the third most common cause of cancer death among males and patients often have progressive and poorly controlled painful bone disease, the limitations that the ineffective measurement of response currently place on effective clinical investigations has important implications for the care of a large number of patients.

Measurement of Primary Prostatic Nodule. There is documented variability in the clinical examination of the prostate and its reporting. Observations by different investigators are often suspect. Sequential digital rectal examination by the same observer can be useful, however, and seem to parallel other measures of response. Occasionally, however, response locally appears to occur at the same time as the bone disease is progressing [23]. The response of local disease if often slow; even patients responding dramatically to estrogen therapy in terms of bone pain, acid phosphatase, etc., will have changes that are minimal at 3 months and often continue to improve between 3 and 6 months. Often more subjective changes in consistency of the prostate and increased urinary stream precede measurable tumor changes, but these are difficult to quantitate. Grids that demonstrate prostatic anatomy in at least two axes are essential for careful documentation of response.

The use of rectal ultrasound has been moderately encouraging [9, 15, 20, 21, 28] in augmenting the clinical examination. Clinically unapparent seminal vesicle involvement was documented by ultrasound in four of ten clinical stage A and B patients and confirmed in radical prostatectomy. Local tumor regression after hormonal therapy

Recent Results in Cancer Research. Vol. 85

could be identified as a decrease in the echogenic dense areas typical of tumor involvement, as well as by a 10%–20% decrease in total gland size [20]. How this correlates with clinical assessment of tumors in unclear, however. Somewhat discouragingly, the technique did not identify progression of local disease with regularity.

Acid Phosphatase. The acid phosphatases are a group of enzymes that are present in all body fluids and tissues. They hydrolyze esters of phosphates at an acid pH. They are predominately lysosomal enzymes found in glandular epithelium. Per unit weight, prostatic tissue has 1,000 times the concentration of any other tissue. Prostatic cancers have less measurable enzyme activity than normal prostate [31].

There are multiple isoenzymes of acid phosphatase. The use of various substrates or the response to various inhibitors of the enzymatic reaction have been used to identify an enzymatic activity largely attributable to the acid phosphatases of prostatic tissues. Disappointingly, this increased specificity of the prostatic acid phosphatase has never translated into augmented clinical utility. The conventional serum acid phosphatase has been shown to be as useful as the more specific enzymatic assay [14].

The degree of initial elevation of acid phosphatase has been shown in most series to have prognostic significance. When patients with bone metastases with elevated serum acid phosphatase are compared to those with normal serum acid phosphatase, the patients with normal serum acid phosphatase are seen to live longer [14]. A single exception was the study of Ishibe et al. [11], where the degree of initial elevation of serum acid phosphatase did not correlate with survival following hormonal therapy. Among patients with elevated serum acid phosphate, the higher the elevation, the worse the survival [2].

The serum acid phosphatase does correlate with other measures of response, although imperfectly. Johnson et al. [12] showed that normalization of serum acid phosphatase correlated with pain relief and reduction of primary tumor mass: In their series, 17 of 91 patients had a 50% or greater reduction of their tumor mass on chemotherapy. Of these 17 patients, 10 (59%) had a normalization of serum acid phosphatase. Of the 74 whose primary cancer did not respond, nine (12%) normalized their serum acid phosphatase. Whether these nine patients did as well as the ten who also had primary tumor reduction is not known. The absolute utility is hampered by any gold standard of response. As a single variable, the reduction or normalization of acid phosphatase correlated doses with improved patient outcome in most series [2, 11].

The various immunologically based tests used for the identification of prostatic acid phosphatase, which have been developed in recent years, have rekindled interest in acid phosphatase as a screening tool. The radioimmune assay (RIA) has been reported to be more effective than the enzymatic assay in screening for early prostate cancer [6]. This has been challenged, though [19, 29]. As a response parameter, however, the (RIA) acid phosphatase has been studied in a limited number of patients [26].

Bone Scan. Bone scintigraphy is the most frequently used clinical test in nuclear medicine. The introduction of $99m_{Tc}$-labeled phosphate [24] and phosphonate compounds [32] was particularly important in improving the sensitivity of scanning. Further, the introduction of whole-body scanning devices has greatly amplified the utility of the $99m_{Tc}$ compounds.

Whole-body scintigraphy is the best method for early detection of bone metastases [16, 22]. This is especially the case in primary tumors such as prostate and breast, which usually produce osteoblastic metastases. With the exception of the rare 'super scan', there are few false negatives in patients who have bone metastases from prostate cancer; further, the bone scan may by grossly abnormal when the skeletal survey is normal and when there is no elevation of alkaline phosphatase or prostatic acid phosphatase.

Recently, there have been a number of approaches to the standardization and, to a lesser extent, the quantitation of changes on bone scans. In breast cancer [4, 7] and prostate cancer [3] a system that maps the abnormalities on a schematized skeleton has been devised. This allows calculation of the percent of bone area involved, and appears to be superior to visual inspection of scans. With this system, progression is identified early, but the identification of early response remains imperfect.

A number of investigators [10, 17] have demonstrated that careful attention to details, including quality control of soft tissue background on scans, improved the qualitative judgements about such scans, and demonstrated the close correlation of such measurements with objective evidence of response, stabilization, or progression. Hardy et al. [8] have suggested an index for monitoring bone scan abnormalities with included evaluation of regions of interest sequentially in patients, and presented three illustrative cases of this methodology.

Nevertheless, metastases to bone remain an area where bone scanning as conventionally employed is relatively insensitive to measure response or progression, particularly over a period of weeks to a few months. Radiographs have been documented to show a further osteoblastic response 44% of the time when the patient is responding unequivocally to treatment [18]. This osteoblastic response to treatment is often mistaken for progression. Once this osteoblastic response occurred in Pollen and Shlaer's series, it usually persisted unchanged in responding patients. Since bone scanning agents will depict increased bone turnover regardless of whether this is due to tumor spread or tumor destruction, the interpretation of bone scan findings must be made in relation to the patient's overall clinical course. Ancillary tests of bone turnover, such as urine hydroxyproline, used in conjunction with other evidence of disease activity, may be helpful in making judgements about tumor response or progression on bone scans [13].

Prognostic Factors for Response and Survival. Prostatic carcinoma has a variable natural history. Although the median survival from time of diagnosis of metastatic disease to death is relatively short (12−18 months in most series), there is a group of patients who can live with metastatic disease up to 5 years and occasionally longer [1]. Table 1 lists the factors, independent of treatment, which have been reported to affect response or survival in prostate cancer. These factors have only been subjected to multivariate analysis in Veterans Administration Cooperative Research Group (VACURG) studies [2]. Thus, some might not independently predict an adverse outcome. Nonetheless, the persistent biologic heterogeneity of these tumors, so well illustrated for localized disease, persists for metastatic disease. Until the effect of chemotherapy is so great as to lessen the importance of these variables, it must be recognized that the comparison of chemotherapeutic agents between nonrandomized studies might relate more to these prognostic factors than to the relative efficacy of the drugs tested.

Partial Response Criteria. Compounding this problem of technical difficulties in assessing response in prostatic cancer is the variable use of this data by different

Table 1. Patient and tumor variables affecting response and/or survival in prostatic cancer

Stage	Group(s) reporting	For hormone therapy	For chemotherapy
Histologic grade	VACURG, NPCP	Yes	No
Progression versus presentation stage D	VACURG, Duke	Yes	No
Urinary obstruction	VACURG	Yes	NS[a]
Initial acid phosphatase	VACURG, Duke	Yes	Yes
Previous radiation	Duke, ECOG, NPCP	NS	Yes/No
Anemia	NPCP, VACURG	Yes	Yes
Performance status	ECOG, VACURG	Yes	Yes
Amount of disease on bone scan	VACURG, Duke	Yes	NS
Abnormal liver scan findings	NPCP, Duke	Yes	Yes
Positive bone marrow biopsy	NPCP	Yes	NS
Age	VACURG, Duke	No	Yes
Severity of bone pain	Duke	NS	Yes

[a] *NS*, not specified or unknown
For other abbreviations see Table 2

Table 2. Partial response criteria [25]

Response sites	Investigator[a]						
	MSKCC	Duke	NPCP	ECOG	SWOG	NCI-VA group	NCOG
Tumor							
↓ 50% measurable area	X	X[b]	X	X	X	X	X
Acid phosphatase							
Return to normal	–	X	X	–	–	–	–
50% reduction	X			X	X	X	X
Alkaline phosphatase							
Return to normal		X	X				
50% reduction	NS[c]			X	X	NS	X
Functional status							
Weight must not significantly decrease	NS	X	X	NS	X	X	X
Performance status must not decrease	NS	X	X	NS	X	X	X
Bones							
Recalcification of lytic bone lesions	NS	X	NS	NS	NS	NS	NS
Concomitant radiation for pain constitutes treatment failure	NS	NS	NS	No	Yes	NS	Yes

[a] *MSKCC*, Memorial-Sloan Kettering Cancer Center; *Duke*, Duke Medical Center; *NPCP*, National Prostatic Cancer Project; *ECOG*, Eastern Cooperative Oncology Group; *SWOG*, Southwest Oncology Group; *NCI-VA group*, National Cancer Institute-Veterans Administration Group; *NCOG*, Northern California Oncology Group

[b] *X*, criteria used by investigator

[c] *NS*, not specified or not known

research groups in the definition of response. This is illustrated in Table 2. Such issues as whether concomitant hormonal therapy is allowed during chemotherapy, the extent of acid phosphatase reduction, etc., may make important differences in the eventual response rate reported.

Stabilization Criteria. The inability to measure disease has led to the incorporation of 'stabilization' in response criteria for prostatic carcinomas treated with systemic agents. The necessity for some measure of progression-free interval is a pragmatic necessity given that more than 80% of patients with metastatic prostatic cancer have only positive bone scans but no soft tissue disease which would be classified 'measurable disease'. Nonetheless, objections have been raised as to the possibility of observer bias in scoring as well as the independent reproducibility of some measurements of stabilization. In addition, it has been suggested that stabilization is simply a reflection of the 'lead time' phenomenon, i.e., that patients who have slower growing tumors are categorized as 'stabilized' but are really unaffected by chemotherapy [30].

Dramatic differences in progression-free interval independent of treatment could be reported depending on the frequency at when the bone scan was performed in otherwise 'stable' patients. Frequent scans might demonstrate asymptomatic progression. Thus it is necessary for large clinical trial groups to define response and progression not in general terms but by the tests used to determine them and the frequency with which they must be performed (i.e., bone scan every 6 months, etc.).

Testicular Carcinoma

For patients treated with chemotherapy for bulky stage II or stage III disease, complete response is the only meaningful outcome, since approximately 70%−90% of patients who enter a complete response will remain continuously disease-free after 2 years. A complete response is defined in testicular carcinoma as complete disappearance of all malignancy. This should be defined by a complete restaging after chemotherapy or the combination of surgery and chemotherapy. In addition to a negative physical examination, this should include reexamination of the retroperitoneal space with a computerized tomographic (CT) scan. It should include repeat whole-lung tomography in all patients who had pulmonary disease or equivocal findings on initial pulmonary tomography. It should include negative alphafetoprotein and BHCG. Reinvestigation of all other sites of initial involvement (liver, brain, etc.) should be undertaken.

It has been recognized that the chemotherapeutic partial response in testicular carcinoma is histologically heterogenous. Residual masses post chemotherapy fall into three distinct groups: (1) fibrosis/necrosis, (2) mature teratoma, and (3) persistent tumor (embryonal carcinoma, immature teratoma, choriocarcinoma, etc.). These correlate with patient outcome [5, 27]. Patients with mature teratoma or fibrosis/necrosis have a prognosis equivalent to those of chemotherapeutic complete response, whereas patients with persistent cancer at second surgery have a worse prognosis. In addition, any one of these histologic findings can be associated with either a complete or incomplete surgical resection. The use of terms like partial response and complete response when applied to the chemotherapy result confer little biologic information. Careful definition of the timing and extent of surgical

intervention in the chemotherapeutic partial responses is still not completely elucidated. A full reporting of status of patients with chemotherapeutic partial response is necessary. One approach is as follows:
(1) Number of evaluable patients with a chemotherapeutic complete response.
(2) Number of patients with residual mass post-chemotherapy
    a) with normal markers,
    b) with residual elevation of markers.
(3) Pathologic outcome
    a) fibrosis/necrosis
       1) complete surgical resection,
       2) incomplete surgical resection,
    b) mature teratoma
       1) complete surgical resection,
       2) incomplete surgical resection,
    c) residual cancer (immature teratoma, embryonal carcinoma, etc.)
       1) complete surgical resection,
       2) incomplete surgical resection.
Each of these should then be related to outcome in terms of relapse-free survival.

Bladder Cancer

For the majority of patients with regionally or distantly metastatic transitional cell carcinoma, the application of conventional response criteria for complete and partial response is adequate. The increased utilization of CT scanning has markedly increased the ability to quantitate response in the retroperitoneum. A group of patients remain with diffuse tumor involvement of the pelvis, where quantitation remains difficult and the time up to progression remains the most useful measure of the utility of chemotherapy.

Renal Cell Carcinoma

Responses to metastatic cancer are infrequent, regardless of the hormonal or chemotherapeutic approach. Investigators searching for any sign of chemotherapeutic activity have tended to be liberal with the definition of response. Often, 25% reductions in tumor size have been classified as a tumor response. Unfortunately, these minimal tumor reductions are subject to considerable observer bias and probably have little biologic meaning. Equally distressing to other investigators, these liberal definitions preclude response comparisons of activity to other solid tumors. Further, many studies do not make any attempt to define response. Other studies score stabilization as a response. In a tumor with such variable natural history, relating stabilization to an effect of treatment is suspect.
Mixed responses are common in renal cell cancer; these are variably recorded as partial response or stabilization; they are rarely reported as a separate category; these mixed responses are virtually never evaluated relative to their effects on patient outcome. Similarly, responses in soft tissue, lung, and bone might be different in terms of frequency, durability, and impact on the patient; yet rarely are sites of response recorded, except in relation to spontaneous regression.

References

1. Bagshaw MA (1978) Radiation therapy for cancer of the prostate. In: Skinner DG, de Kernion JB (eds) Genitourinary cancer. Saunders, New York, p 358
2. Byar DP (1977) VACURG studies on prostatic cancer and its treatment. In: Tannenbaum M (ed) Urologic pathology: the prostate. Lea & Febiger, Philadelphia, pp 241–267
3. Citrin DL, Cohen AI, Harberg J, Schlise S, Hougen C, Benson (1981) Systemic treatment of advanced prostatic cancer: development of a new system for defining response. J Urol 125: 224–227
4. Citrin DL, Hougen C, Zweibel W, Schlise S, Pruitt B, Ershler W, Davis TE, Harberg J, Cohen AI (1981) The use of serial bone scans in assessing response of bone metastases to systemic treatment. Cancer 47: 680–685
5. Einhorn LH, Williams SD, Mandelbaum I, Donohur JP (1981) Surgical resection in disseminated testicular cancer following chemotherapeutic cytoreduction. Cancer 48: 904–908
6. Foti AG, Cooper JF, Hershman H, Malvaez RR (1977) Detection of prostatic cancer by solid-phase radioimmunoassay of serum prostatic acid phosphatase. N Engl J Med 297: 1357–1362
7. Galasko CSB, Doyle FM (1972) The response to therapy of skeletal metastases from mammary cancer: assessment of scintigraphy. Br J Surg 59: 85–88
8. Hardy JG, Kulatilake AE, Wastie ML (1980) An index for monitoring bone metastases from carcinoma of the prostate. Br J Radiol 53: 869–873
9. Henneberry M, Carter MF, Neiman HL (1979) Estimation of prostatic size by suprapubic ultrasonography. J Urol 121: 615–616
10. Hovsepian JA, Byar DP and the VACURG (1978) Quantitative radiology of responses to endocrine therapy in stage 4 adenocarcinoma of the prostate. Proc AACR and ASCO 19: 307
11. Ishibe T, Usui T, Nihira H (1974) Prognostic usefulness of serum acid phosphatase levels in carcinoma of the prostate. J Urol 112: 237–240
12. Johnson DE, Scott WW, Gibbons RP, Prout GR, Schmidt JD, Murphy GP (1976) Clinical significance of serum acid phosphatase levels in advanced prostatic carcinoma. Urology 8: 123–126
13. Mooppan MMU, Wax SH, Kim H, Wang JC, Tobin MS (1980) Urinary hydroxyproline excretion as a marker of osseous metastasis in carcinoma of the prostate. J Urol 123: 694–696
14. Murphy GP, Reynoso G, Kenny GM, Gaeta JF (1969) Comparison of total and prostatic fraction serum acid phosphatase levels in patients with differentiated and undifferentiated prostatic carcinoma. Cancer 23: 1309–1314
15. Peeling WB, Griffiths GJ, Evans KT, Roberts EE (1979) Diagnosis and staging of prostatic cancer by transrectal ultrasonography. A preliminary study. Br J Urol 51: 565–569
16. Pistenma DA, McDougall IR, Kriss JP (1975) Screening for bone metastases. Are only scans necessary? JAMA 231: 46–50
17. Pollen JJ, Gerber K, Ashburn WL, Schmidt JD (1981) Nuclear bone imaging in metastatic cancer of the prostate. Cancer 47: 2585–2594
18. Pollen JJ, Shlaer (1979) Osteoblastic response to successful treatment of metastatic cancer of the prostate. AJR 132: 927–931
19. Quinones GR, Rohner TJ, Drago JR, Demers LM (1981) Will prostatic acid phosphatase determination by radioimmunoassay increase the diagnosis of early prostatic cancer? J Urol 125: 361–364
20. Resnick MI, Willard JW, Boyce WH (1980) Transrectal ultrasonography in the evaluation of patients with prostatic carcinoma. J Urol 124: 482–484
21. Resnick MI, Willard JW, Boyce WH (1981) Ultrasonic evaluation of the prostatic nodule. J Urol 120: 86–89

22. Shafer RB, Reinke DB (1977) Contribution of the bone scan, serum acid and alkaline phosphatase, and the radiographic bone survey to the management of newly-diagnosed carcinoma of the prostate. Clin Nucl Med 2: 200–203
23. Slack NH, Mittelman A, Brady MF, Murphy GP (1980) The importance of the stable category for chemotherapy treated patients with advanced and relapsing prostate cancer. Cancer 46: 2393–2402
24. Subramanian G, McAfee JG, Bell EG, Blair RJ, O'Mara RE (1972) 99m$_{Tc}$-labeled polyphosphate as a skeletal imaging agent. Radiology 102: 701–704
25. Torti FM, Carter SK (1980) The chemotherapy of prostatic carcinoma. Ann Intern Med 92: 681–689
26. Vihko P, Lukkarinen, Kontturi M, Vihko R (1981) Effectiveness of radioimmunoassay of human prostate-specific acid phosphatase in the diagnosis and follow-up of therapy in prostatic carcinoma. Cancer Res 41: 1180–1183
27. Vugrin D, Whitmore WF, Sogani PC, Bains M, Herr HW, Golbey RB (1981) Combined chemotherapy and surgery in treatment of advanced germ-cell tumors. Cancer 47: 2228–2231
28. Wantanabe H, Igari D, Tanahasi Y, Harada K, Saitoh M (1975) Development and application of new equipment for transrectal ultrasonography. J Clin Ultrasound 2: 91–98
29. Watson R, Tang DB (1980) The predictive value of prostatic acid phosphatase as a screening test for prostatic cancer. N Engl J Med 303: 497–499
30. Yagoda A, Watson RC, Natale RB, Barzell W, Sogani P, Grabstald H, Whitmore WF (1979) A critical analysis of response criteria in patients with prostatic cancer treated with cis-diamminedichloride platinum II. Cancer 44: 1553–1562
31. Yam LT (1974) Clinical significance of the human acid phosphatases. Am J Med 56: 604–616
32. Yano Y, McRae J, Van Dyke DC, Anger HO (1973) Technetium-99m-labeled stannous ethane-l-hydroxy-1 1-diphosphonate: a new bone scanning agent. J Nucl Med 14: 73

Prostatic Cancer Chemotherapy

F. M. Torti

Division of Medical Oncology, Stanford University Medical Center, Palo Alto, CA, USA

Introduction

Each year, 50,000 new cases of prostatic carcinoma are diagnosed in the United States. It is estimated that 85% have regional or distant metastatic disease at the time of diagnosis. Thus, the management of metastatic disease is a major therapeutic problem for the urologist, radiation therapist, and medical oncologist.

This chapter will not review in detail the literature on the hormonal treatment of prostatic cancer. Instead, the current treatment approach at the conjoint genitourinary oncology clinic at Stanford University Medical Center for those patients with metastatic prostate cancer to bone is presented in Table 1. It illustrates one approach to the standardization of conventional therapy of advanced disease.

This general treatment plan takes into account data from the Veterans Administration Cooperative Research Group (VACURG), suggesting there is no benefit to initial treatment of asymptomatic metastatic disease in most patients [3–5]. The approximately equal therapeutic efficacy of diethylstilbestrol (DES) versus orchiectomy is recognized, and patient preference and medical contraindications to estrogens are the factors that influence the choice of estrogen therapy or orchiectomy. It is recognized that these treatments are palliative and as such all modalities will be utilized in most patients.

The sequence of hormonal and chemotherapeutic maneuvers in Table 1 is dependent upon the anticipated results and the anticipated morbidity. It is felt that the first hormonal manuever is likely to give a response to patients with symptomatic metastatic disease in 60%–90% of cases. Since the cardiovascular safety of doses greater than 1 mg has not been convincingly demonstrated, 1 mg diethylstilbestrol is chosen [42]. Chemotherapy is generally superior to secondary hormonal maneuvers in prostatic cancer in palliative response as well as survival, and is utilized next in the sequence [37]. It is important to recognize that some patients will respond to higher dose DES, particularly when the testosterone is not adequately suppressed on 1 mg. Lack of testosterone suppression on higher doses than 3 mg usually means lack of patient compliance to chronic estrogen use.

Low-dose breast irradiation (900–1,200 rad in three to four daily treatments) is routinely administered prior to DES, and has been shown to reduce gynecomastia [12]. As noted in Table 1, palliative irradiation is used to delay systemic therapy when possible. It is important for the clinician to recognize, however, the pattern of decreasing intervals between palliative radiation treatments as a sign of generalized disease progression, and to utilize systemic therapy when this occurs.

Recent Results in Cancer Research. Vol. 85
© Springer-Verlag Berlin · Heidelberg 1983

Table 1. Current treatment approach at Stanford University Medical Center for patients with metastatic prostate cancer to bone

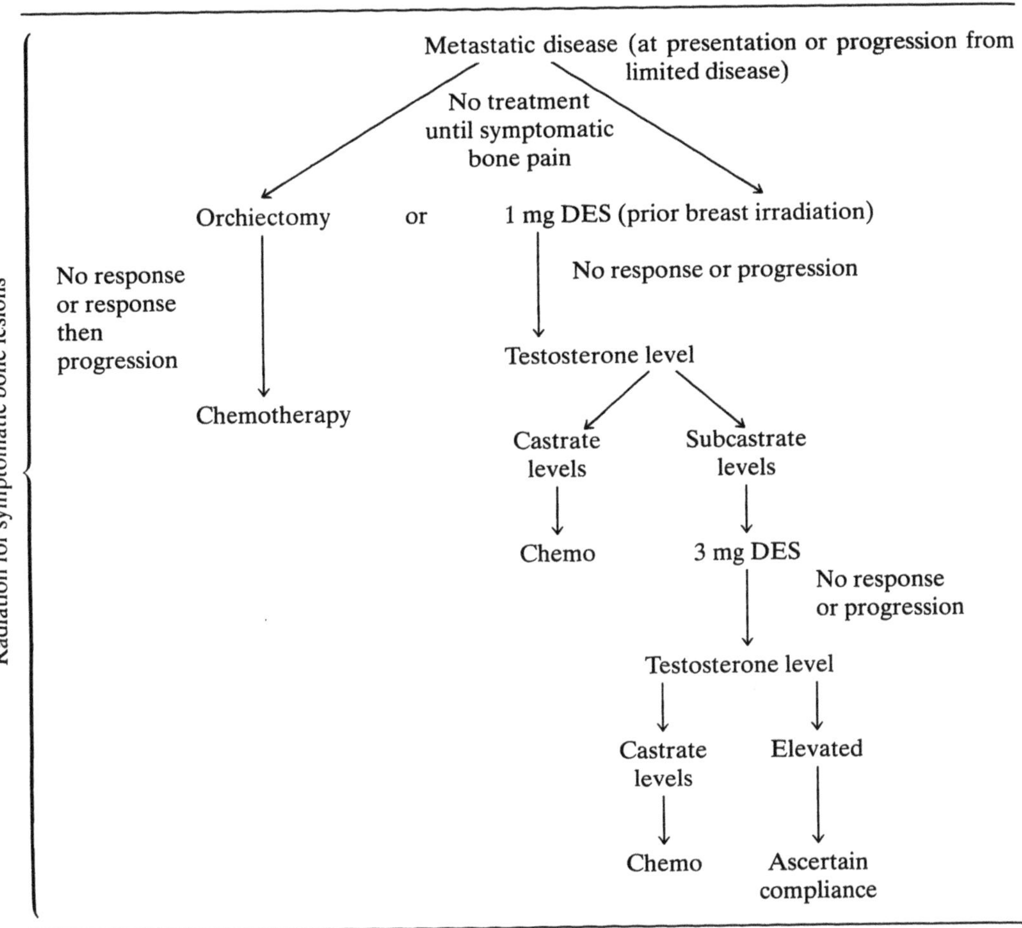

General Principles in the Treatment of Patients With Metastatic Disease

There are a number of principles of treatment of prostatic cancer that are not common to most other neoplastic diseases and which should be mentioned in the context of any discussion of advanced disease management.

1) Time for response to hormonal maneuver: This has not been well studied. It appears that improvement in painful bone lesions usually occurs within 6 weeks in patients who eventually have a response; changes in the palpable local tumor usually are evident in 3 months, but continued response can be documented for at least 6 months. Trials of chemotherapeutic agents should incorporate the possibility of slow response into their design. Judgements about response should not be made before 12 weeks.

2) Short-term variability of painful lesions: Patients with bone pain from prostatic carcinoma undergo changes in the amount of pain and, therefore, in the narcotic

requirement for reasons other than treatment response or progression. Thus, skeletal trauma of a minor degree, musculoskeletal strains, etc., all appear transiently to exacerbate pain in already painful sites of metastatic disease. Protocols should not be designed to score either pain response or progression based on improving or worsening symptoms over the time period of a few weeks. The trend over 2–3 months is required to make a reasonable judgement of symptomatic response or progression.

3) Diffuse bone tenderness indicates need for systemic treatment: Among the patients evaluated prior to palliative radiation therapy, a subset has emerged where a telescoping series of palliative treatments can be predicted, probably warranting early systemic intervention. These are the patients with one or a few sites of symptomatic bone pain, but who have on examination a diffuse tenderness to palpation. These patients in our experience will develop other symptomatic sites in such a short interval that systemic treatment is warranted.

Chemotherapeutic Agents

Prior to 1973, the number of chemotherapeutic trials of prostate cancer had been few (Table 2). Almost none were randomized comparisons. Many reports included a few patients from broad drug-oriented phase II studies, where patients with prostatic carcinoma usually do not have adequate evaluation. The National Prostate Cancer Project (NPCP) has provided the leadership in the large cooperative trials in prostate cancer, which is necessary for the evaluation of new agents in this disease. Other national and regional cooperative groups and large institutions have also begun to place patients on randomized protocols, including the Eastern Cooperative Oncology Group, the Uro-Oncology Research Group, the Mayo Clinic, the Western Cancer Study Group, the Northern California Oncology Group, and others.

Table 3 lists response rates for patients with metastatic prostatic carcinoma. Although there is an occasional report of patients treated initially with chemotherapy for metastatic disease, this table confines itself to patients treated after failure of at least

Table 2. Chemotherapy agents prior to 1973[a, b]

	No. treated	No. responses
Alanine mustard	29	4
BCNU[c]	8	1
Cyclophosphamide	34	4
5-Fluorouracil	39	10
Methorexate	24	3
Mithramycin	21	1
Vincristine	12	1
FUDR[d]	8	3

[a] Only agents studied in more than seven adequately treated patients
[b] Personal communication, SK Carter
[c] *BCNU*, 1,3-bis(2-chloroethyl)-l-nitrosourea
[d] *FUDR*, 5-fluoro-2'-deoxyuridine

Table 3. Overall response rate for single agents in prostatic carcinoma in patients failing hormonal therapy

	Response includes stabilization			Response excludes stabilization		
	Patients no.	Responses no.	(%)	Patients no.	Responses no.	(%)
5-fluorouracil	62	26	(42)	48	5	(10)
Cyclophosphamide	136	52	(38)	–	–	
Doxorubicin	–	–		83	19	(23)
Cisplatin	–	–		70	15	(21)
Dacarbazine (DTIC)	23	9	(39)	–	–	
Procarbazine	21	3	(14)	–	–	
Lomustine (CCNU)	9	1	(11)	10	4	(40)
Melphalan	–	–		15	1	(7)
Streptozocin	38	12	(32)	–	–	
Estramustine	108	50	(46)	319	56	(18)
Prednimustine	–	–		23	3	(13)
Vincristine	34	5	(15)	–	–	
Hydroxyurea	28	4	(15)	–	–	
m-AMSA	15	7	(47)	–	–	
MeCCNU	27	8	(30)			

one, but usually multiple, hormonal therapies. Radiation therapy for pain control in localized sites of bone metastases has been utilized prior to chemotherapy in most patients in this table.

Response rates are divided into those that include and those that exclude 'stabilization' in the definition of tumor response. Even this division implies a degree of reporting homogeneity that is not present, as shown in Table 2, Chap. 3, which illustrates the different definitions of partial response utilized in clinical trials. In addition, the route and dose of drug administered is not consistent even for commonly utilized drugs (Table 7). Nonetheless, Adriamycin, cyclophosphamide and perhaps estramustine, dacarbazine (DTIC), and cisplatin have activity in this disease. Other agents, such as lomustine (CCNU) and m-AMSA, have not been adequately evaluated.

Cyclophosphamide

Cyclophosphamide has been tested in a randomized trial against both 5-fluorouracil (5-FU) and placebo in one study of the NPCP [36–38], and against DTIC and procarbazine in another [34]. In the first study, chemotherapy was shown superior to standard treatment in terms of pain relief, time to progression, and objective responses. Patients appeared well matched for prognostic factors that may affect outcome in advanced prostatic cancer (functional status, age, histologic grade, etc.). It appeared to the authors that cyclophosphamide was superior to 5-FU in terms of number of partial regressions and number of crossover responses; these differences were small, however. Cyclophosphamide was chosen as the standard drug against which to test new agents.

Table 4. Cyclophosphamide in metastatic prostatic cancer (patients failing hormonal therapy)

	Investigator	No. evaluable	Response includes stabilization (%)	Response excludes stabilization (%)	Reference no.
Cyclophosphamide alone	See text	136	38	–	
Cyclophosphamide in combination:					
Cyclophosphamide + 5-FU	Mayo Clinic	18	–	11	[9]
Cyclophosphamide + 5-FU	Roswell Park	13	65	–	[23]
Cyclophosphamide + 5-FU + MTX[a]	Bowman Gray	15	53	–	[28]

[a] *MTX*, methotrexate

Table 5. Doxorubicin in metastatic prostatic carcinoma (patients failing hormonal therapy)

	Investigator	No. evaluable	Response includes stabilization (%)	Response excludes stabilization (%)	Reference no.
Doxorubicin alone	See text	83	–	23	
Doxorubicin in combination:					
Doxorubicin + cyclophosphamide	Wayne State	15	7	–	[14, 15]
Doxorubicin + cyclophosphamide	NCI-VA	22	50	32	[13]
Doxorubicin + cyclophosphamide	Roswell Park	20	69	–	[23]
Doxorubicin + cyclophosphamide + 5-FU	Smalley	29	69	–	[39]
Doxorubicin + cyclophosphamide + 5-FU	Western Group	12	50	–	[6]
Doxorubicin + cyclophosphamide + 5-FU	Soloway	21	81	–	[40]
Doxorubicin + cyclophosphamide + cisplatinum	Wayne State	16	63	–	[1]
Doxorubicin + cyclophosphamide + methotrexate	Boston University	12	75	–	[41]
Doxorubicin + cyclophosphamide + BCNU	Southeast Group	27	–	26	[33]
Doxorubicin + 5-FU + mitomycin C	Logothetis	32	–	62	[18, 19]
Doxorubicin + platinum	Mt. Sinai	17	–	53	[32]

Cyclophosphamide was used again by the NPCP in their studies numbers 300 [35] and 500 [17] with a lower response rate. This difference might be due to factors of patient selection, although this is not completely explained. In the NPCP study number 300 DTIC was also shown to have activity roughly comparable to cyclophosphamide; procarbazine appeared inferior, but it was difficult to deliver full doses due to drug toxicity. In study number 500 methyl-chloroethyl-cyclohexy-nitrosourea (MeCCNU) had about equal efficacy to cyclophosphamide, but was more toxic [17].

Table 3 lists the response rates for cyclophosphamide in combination, compared to the reports of single agent activity. Although the response rates appear higher for combinations, the single randomized study of cyclophosphamide versus combination Rx showed no differences in response or survival (see Table 6) [28].

Table 6. Randomized trials of single-agent vs combination chemotherapy in metastatic prostate carcinoma

	Group	Conclusion	Reference no.
R< Adriamycin / 5-FU + cyclophosphamide	Mayo Clinic	No diff.	[9]
R< 5-FU / 5-FU + cyclophosphamide + doxorubicin	Southeast Oncology Group	No diff.	[39]
R< Cyclophosphamide / Cyclophosphamide + doxorubicin + 5-FU	Western Group	No diff.	[6]
R< Vincristine / Estramustine / Vincristine + estramustine	National Prostatic Cancer Project	No diff.	[40]
R< Cyclophosphamide / Cyclophosphamide + methotrexate + 5-FU	Bowman Gray	No diff.	[28]
R< Prednimustine / Prednimustine + estramustine	National Prostatic Cancer Project	No diff.	[26]

Table 7. Dosage of chemotherapy in selected studies

Chemotherapy Doses[a] Investigator Study Groups	Adria-mycin	Cyclo-phospha-mide	5-Fluoro-uracil	Estra-mustine	Strepto-zotocin	DTIC	Procar-bazine
NPCP		1 gm/m^2/ q3wk	600 mg/m^2 qlwk	200 mg/m^2 po TID	500 mg/m^2 qDX5 q6wK	200 mg/m^2 qDX5 q4wk	100 mg/m^2 qDX21d q6wk
Mayo Clinic	60 mg/m^2 q3wkX2 then q4w	150 mg/m^2 X5d q5wk	300 mg/m^2 qdX5d q5wk				
NCI-VA			600 mg/m^2 qlwkX4, then 750 mg/m^2 qwk				
ECOG	60 mg/m^2 q3wk 40 mg/m^2 q3wk		600 mg/m^2 qlwk or 400 mg/m^2 qlwk				
Roswell Park	40 mg/m^2 q3wk	4 mg/kg qDX5 q4wk	8 mg/kg qDX5 q4wk	15 mg/Rg po qD			
Wayne State	40 mg/m^2 q3wk X 5 30 mg/m^2	500 mg/m^2 q3wk or 400 mg/m^2 q3wk					
Boston U.	40 mg/m^2 q3wk	600 mg/m^2 q3wk					
Uro-Oncology Group			500 po				
NCI-VA	30 mg/m^2 d1 + 8	100 mg/m^2 po qD1−14					
Yale			600 mg/m^2 qlwk	24 mg/kg/D po			
Perloff et al.	50−60 mg q3−4wk						
Merrin							
Yagoda							
Western Group	30−50 mg/m^2 IV D1	800−1200 mg/m^2 q3wk	400−500 mg/m^2 D1 + D8				

[a] IV unless noted

CCNU	Metho-trexate	Mephalan	Vinchris-tine	Pred-nisone	Predni-mustine	Cis-platinum	Hydroxy-urea	MeCCNU
							3 g/m^2 po qdX3	175 mg/m^2 q6wks
130 mg/m^2 po								
						25 mg/m^2 po qD		
	15 mg/m^2 po q9, 13, 16, 20							
	25 mg po q7d	2 mg po qd	1 mg qwkX4 q4mo	40 mg po taper to 10 mg po				
						50 mg/m^2 q2–4wk		
						1 mg/kg qlwkX6, then q3wk		
						50–70 mg/m^2 q3wk		

Adriamycin

Adriamycin has been studied in a large number of patients in prostatic cancer. A dose-response effect was shown for prostatic cancer in a Southwest Oncology Group (SWOG) study. For good-risk patients, the response rate for adriamycin administered every 3 weeks was 3/10 patients at 75 mg/m^2, 2/4 patients at 60 mg/m^2, 0/5 patients at 45 mg/m^2. Poor-risk patients, defined in the study as patients with entry WBC between 3,000 and 5,000/mm^3 or platelet count between 100,000 and 150,000/mm^3 or abnormal liver function tests, had 0/19 responses, although a number of these patients were treated at subtherapeutic doses of Adriamycin (25 mg/m^2 every 3−4 weeks) [31]. Adriamycin was clearly superior to 5-FU in a study of the ECOG [7, 8].
Table 5 lists the multiple combination chemotherapies reported that include Adriamycin. Response rates vary widely; no definite evidence of superiority emerges over single-agent treatment.

Estramustine

Estramustine phosphate (an ester of nitrogen mustard and estradiol) has been studied widely in Europe and to a lesser extent in the United States. A randomized study by the NPCP [27] demonstrated that the response rate to estramustine was similar (30%) to streptozotocin (32%), but superior to standard therapy (19%). However, the responses were more durable with estramustine (45 weeks) than with streptozoticin (31 weeks) or standard therapy (30 weeks). This study was conducted in a group of patients who had received extensive prior radiation therapy; although any disease appeared to stabilize, none had a partial response. When used as first hormonal therapy, estramustine has had impressive response rates but does not appear to be better than estrogen alone. Even at low doses, estramustine was demonstrated to reduce the serum testosterone [11]. In patients who failed estrogen therapy, some response rates were in the 50% ranges [2, 29, 30], but most were in the 25% range [10, 16, 24, 25]. Used in combination with methotrexate and cisplatin, four of nine patients had an objective response and two others a subjective response [20].
In patients who fail one estrogenic therapy for prostatic carcinoma, responses to other estrogen compounds have been reported − whether estramustine is qualitatively or quantitatively different from standard hormonal treatments in terms of its ability to generate secondary hormonal response remains to be demonstrated.

Cisplatin

Cisplatin has been utilized with variable results in metastatic prostatic carcinoma. Merrin et al. have reported [22, 23] that 13 of 45 patients obtained an objective response and six other patients 'stabilized' their disease when treated with cisplatin 1 mg/kg for 6 weeks then every 3 weeks until relapse. Yagoda et al. [43] using only patients with measurable tumor nodules, found a 12% (3/25) objective response rate, which could have been reported as a response rate of 4%−23%, depending on the response criteria used by various investigative groups. The emphasis on the unusual measured metastasis may have selected out a biologically distinct subgroup of prostate cancer. The utility of cisplatin in metastatic prostatic cancer is still uncertain.

Some important benchmarks by which we judge utility of cancer treatment are not readily available in prostatic carcinoma; this has discouraged some investigators from studying this disease; it has prompted others to express either undue pessimism or optimism about the utility of chemotherapy of this disease. It is clear, however, that a number of chemotherapeutic agents in prostatic carcinoma are useful to the physician concerned with palliation of his patients: A variety of these agents will cause substantive pain relief in 30%−60% of patients; objective response rates exceeding 25% of patients have been reported with a number of these drugs. Responses tend to be of short duration, 4−8 months; this is not dramatically different, however, from chemotherapeutic regimens in other solid tumors.

References

1. Al-Sarraf M (1980) Combination of cytoxan, adriamycin and cis-platinum (CAP) in patients with advanced prostatic cancer. Proc AACR and ASCO 21: 198
2. Andersson L, Edsmyr F, Jonsson G, Konyves I (1977) Estramustine phosphate therapy in carcinoma of the prostate. In: Grundmann E, Vahlensieck W (eds) Tumors of the male genital system. Springer, Berlin Heidelberg New York, pp 73−77 (Recent Results in Cancer Research, vol 60)
3. Arduino L, Bailar JL, Becker L et al. (1967) Carcinoma of the prostate treatment comparison. J Urol 98: 516−522
4. Arduino L, Bailar JL, Becker L, et al. (1967) Treatment and survival of patients with cancer of the prostate. Surg Gynecol Obstet 124: 1011−1017
5. Byar DP (1977) VACURG studies on prostatic carcinoma. In: Tannenbaum M (ed) Urologic pathology: the prostate, Lea and Febiger, Philadelphia, p 241
6. Chlebowski RT, Hestorff R, Sardoff L, Weiner J, Bateman JR (1978) Cyclophosphamide (NSC 26271) versus the combination of adriamycin (NSC 123127), 5-fluorouracil (NSC 19893), and cyclophosphamide in the treatment of metastatic prostatic cancer. A randomized trial. Cancer 42: 2546−2552
7. DeWys WD, Bauer M, Colsky J, Cooper RA, Creech R, Carbone PP (1977) Comparative trial of adriamycin and 5-fluorouracil in advanced prostatic cancer-Progress report. Cancer Treat Rep 61: 325−328
8. DeWys DW, Begg CB (1978) Comparison of adriamycin (ADRIA) and 5-fluorouracil (5 FU) in advanced prostatic cancer. Proc AACR and ASCO 19: 331
9. Eagan RT, Hahn RG, Myers RP (1976) Adriamycin (NSC 127127) versus 5-fluorouracil (NSC 19893) and cyclophosphamide (NSC 26271) in the treatment of metastatic prostate cancer. Cancer Treat Rep 60: 115−117
10. Fossa SD, Miller A (1976) Treatment of advanced carcinoma of the prostate with estramustine phosphate. J Urol 115: 406−408
11. Fritjofsson A, Norlen BJ, Hogberg B, Rajalakshmi, Cekan SZ, Doczfalusy E (1981) Hormonal effects of different doses of estramustine phosphate (estracyT) in patients with prostatic carcinoma. Scand J Urol Nephrol 15: 37−44
12. Gagnon JF, Moss WT, Stevens KR (1979) Pre-estrogen breast irradiation for patients with carcinoma of the prostate: A critical review. J Urol 121: 182−184
13. Ihde DC, Bunn PA, Cohen MH, Dunnick NR, Eddy JL, Minna JD (1980) Effective treatment of hormonally-unresponsive metastatic carcinoma of the prostate with adriamycin and cyclophosphamide. Cancer 45: 1300−1310
14. Izbicki RM, Amer MH, Al-Sarraf M (1979) Combination of adriamycin and cyclophosphamide in the treatment of metastatic prostatic carcinoma: A Phase II study. Cancer Treat Rep 63: 999−1001

15. Izbicki RM, Amer M, Al-Sarraf M (1978) A prospective study of a combination of adriamycin and cytoxan in the treatment of patients with advanced prostatic cancer. Proc Am Assoc Cancer Res Am Soc Clin Oncol 19:312 (abstract)
16. Lindberg B (1972) Treatment of rapidly progressing prostatic carcinoma with estracyt. J Urol 108:303–306
17. Leoning SA, Scott WW, deKernion J, Gibbons RP, Johnson DE, Pontes JE, Prout GR, Schmidt JD, Soloway MS, Chu TM, Gaeta JF, Slack NH, Murphy GP (1981) A comparison of hydroxyurea, methyl-chloroethyl-cyclohexy-nitrosourea and cyclophosphamide in patients with advanced carcinoma of the prostate. J Urol 125:812–816
18. Logothetis C, von Eschenbach A, Samuels M, Haynie TP, Johnson DE (1981) Doxorubicin, mitomycin-C, 5-fluorouracil (DMF) in the therapy of hormonal resistant adenocarcinoma of the prostate. Proc AACR and ASCO 22:462
19. Logothetis CJ, von Eschenbach AC, Samuels ML, Trindade A, Johnson DE (1982) Doxorubicin, Mitomycin, and 5-FU (DMF) in the treatment of hormone-resistant stage D prostate cancer: a preliminary report. Cancer Treat Rep 66:57–63
20. Madajewicz S, Catane R, Mittelman A, Wajsman Z, Murphy GP (1980) Chemotherapy of advanced, hormonally resistant prostatic carcinoma. Oncology 37:53–56
21. Merrin C (1978) Treatment of advanced carcinoma of the prostate (stage D) with infusion of cis-diamminedichloroplatinum (II NSC 119875): a pilot study. J Urol 119:522–524
22. Merrin CE, Beckley A (1979) The treatment of estrogen-resistant stage D carcinoma of the prostate with cis-diamminedichloroplatinum. Urology 13:267–272
23. Merrin C, Etra W, Wajsman Z, Baumgartner G, Murphy G (1976) Chemotherapy of advanced carcinoma of the prostate with 5-fluorouracil, cyclophosphamide, and adriamycin. J Urol 115:86–88
24. Mittelman A, Shukla SK, Welvaar TK, Murphy GP (1975) Oral estramustine phosphate in the treatment of advanced stage D carcinoma of the prostate. Cancer Chemother Rep 59:219–223
25. Mittelman A, Shukla SK, Murphy GP (1976) Extended therapy of stage D carcinoma of the prostate with oral estramustine phosphate. J Urol 115:409–412
26. Murphy GP, Gibbons RP, Johnson DE et al. (1979) The use of estramustine and prednimustine versus prednimustine alone in advanced metastatic prostatic cancer patients who have received prior irradiation. J Urol 121:763–765
27. Murphy GP, Gibbons RP, Johnson DE (1977) A comparison of estramustine phosphate and streptozotocin in patients with advanced prostatic carcinoma who have had extensive irradiation. J Urol 118:288–291
28. Muss HB, Howard V, Richards F, White DR, Jackson DV, Cooper MR, Stuart JJ, Resnick MI, Brodkin R, Spurr CL (1981) Cyclophosphamide versus cyclophosphamide, methotrexate, and 5-fluorouracil in advanced prostatic cancer: a randomized trial. Cancer 47:1949–1953
29. Nagel R, Kollin SP (1976) Treatment of advanced carcinoma of the prostate with estracyt. In: Marberger H (ed) Prostatic disease. Liss, New York, pp 267–283
30. Nagel R, Kollin CP (1977) Treatment of advanced carcinoma of the prostate with estramustine phosphate. Br J Urol 49:73–79
31. O'Bryan RM, Baker LH, Gottlieb JE et al. (1977) Dose response evaluation of adriamycin in human neoplasia. Cancer 39:1940–1948
32. Perloff M, Ohnuma T, Holland JF, Kennedy BJ, Mills RC (1977) Adriamycin (ADM) and diamminedichloroplatinum (DDP) in advanced prostatic carcinoma (PC). Proc Am Assoc Cancer Res Am Soc Clin Oncol 18:333 (abstract)
33. Presant CA, Van Amburg A, Klahr C, Metter GE (1980) Chemotherapy of advanced prostatic cancer with adriamycin, BCNU, and cyclophosphamide. Cancer 46:2389–2392
34. Schmidt JD, Scott WW, Gibbons RP et al. (1979) Comparison of procarbazine, imidazole-carboxamide and cyclophosphamide in relapsing patients with advanced carcinoma of the prostate. J Urol 121:185–189

35. Schmidt JD, Johnson DE, Scott WW, Gibbons RP, Prout GR, Murphy GP (1976) Chemotherapy of advanced prostatic cancer: evaluation of response parameters. Urology 7: 602–610
36. Scott W, Johnson DE, Schmidt JE et al. (1976) Chemotherapy of advanced prostatic carcinoma with cyclophosphamide or 5-fluorouracil: results of first national randomized study. J Urol 114: 909–911
37. Scott WW, Gibbons RP, Johnson DE et al. (1975) Comparison of 5-fluorouracil (NSC-019893) and cyclophosphamide (NSC-026271) in patients with advanced carcinoma of the prostate. Cancer Chemother Rep 59: 195–201
38. Scott WW, Gibbons RP, Johnson DE et al. (1976) The continued evaluation of the effects of chemotherapy in patients with advanced carcinoma of the prostate. J Urol 116: 211–213
39. Smalley RV, Bartolucci AA, Hemstreet G, Hester M (1981) A phase II evaluation of a 3-drug combination of cyclophosphamide, doxorubicin and 5-fluorouracil and or 5-fluorouracil in patients with advanced bladder carcinoma or stage D prostatic carcinoma. J Urol 125: 191–195
40. Soloway MS, de Kernion JB, Gibbons RP, Johnson DE, Leoning SA, Pontes JE, Prout GR, Schmidt JD, Scott WW, Chu TM, Gaeta JF, Slack NH, Murphy GP (1981) Comparison of estramustine phosphate and vincristine alone or in combination for patients with advanced hormone refractory, previously irradiated carcinoma of the prostate. J Urol 125: 664–667
41. Straus MJ, Parmelee J, Olsson C, De Vere White R (1978) Cytoxan, adriamycin and methotrexate (CAM) therapy of stage D prostate cancer. Proc Am Assoc Cancer Res Am Soc Clin Oncol 19: 314 (abstract)
42. Torti FM, Carter SK (1980) The chemotherapy of prostatic adenocarcinoma. Ann Intern Med 92: 681–689
43. Yagoda A, Watson RC, Natale RB, Barzell W, Sogani P, Grabstald H, Whitmore WF (1979) A critical analysis of response criteria in patients with prostatic cancer treated with cis-diamminedichloride platinum II. Cancer 44: 1553–1562

The Management of Testicular Cancer

S. K. Carter

Northern California Cancer Program, P.O. Box 10144, Palo Alto, CA 94303, USA

Introduction

Testicular neoplasms are rare tumors that account for only about 1% of all cancers occurring in males and have an average annual incidence of about 2.3 per 100,000 males in the English-speaking population [19, 32]. Nevertheless, these tumors have a dramatic impact because they occur predominantly in young men. Excluding leukemias and lymphomas, testicular tumors are the leading cause of lethal cancer in men from 25 to 34 years of age [57].

The treatment of malignant testicular tumors, with the possible exception of classic seminoma, is a topic of controversy produced largely by differences of opinion concerning their histologic classification and evaluation of the extent of tumor spread at the time of initial diagnosis. Some resolution of these diagnostic problems is of paramount importance in selecting therapeutic approaches and estimating prognosis in these tumors.

The incidence of testicular cancer shows two age peaks. The highest rate in the United States is seen for white men aged 30–34 years. There is a second peak, but not as high, in older men. Recent data also suggest a peak in early childhood for whites. In black men under the age of 65 years the incidence is very low but after the age of 65 years both blacks and whites have similar rates [21].

When pathologic subtypes are examined, the proportions of embryonal carcinoma and teratocarcinoma decrease. It is this latter nonseminatous group of histologies that account for the peak in early adulthood, which is not observed in most other cancer sites. The relative deficit of testicular cancer among young adult black men is greatest for the histologies other than seminoma [62].

The National Cancer Survey results indicate that the incidence of testicular cancer in blacks dropped nearly 50% between 1947–1948 and 1969–1971 [22]. On the other hand, over the middle third of this century there have been small increases in both incidence and mortality in whites. Age-specific data indicate that this rise has occurred primarily among young adults [74].

The most important risk factor identified for the development of testicular malignancy is undescended testes, although clear delineation of the magnitude of the risk is lacking. In young adults there appears to be a tenfold increase of risk in this situation. The association of risk with maldescent is stronger for seminoma than for their histologic types. Surgical correction of an undescended testicle will reduce the risk, indicating that the undescended testicle itself is the causal factor rather than maldescent and malignancy being due to a common cause. This question, however, is not fully resolved [63].

Recent Results in Cancer Research, Vol. 85
© Springer-Verlag Berlin · Heidelberg 1983

Another suggested risk factor is inguinal hernia in children [48] or young adults [63]. The relative risk has been suggested to be threefold. Hernia tends to coexist with undescended testis. At present it is uncertain whether this association explains the link between hernia and testicular cancer [63].

More than half of testis tumors are initially misdiagnosed as epididymitis. In every large series there exists patients whose diagnosis was delayed while antibiotic trials were undertaken.

The natural history of testicular cancer begins usually as small intratesticular lesions. Most will ultimately replace the majority of the testicular parenchyma. The mass will spread locally to the rete testis, epididymis, and the spermatic cord. The tunica albuginea forms a natural barrier but the tumor may even rarely invade this natural barrier and penetrate into scrotal fat.

The most common initial clinical manifestation will be a mass in the testis. All testicular masses must be considered malignant unless proven otherwise. In some choriocarcinomas, endocrine symptoms and gyneomastia may be the first manifestations.

Prognostic Variables

Histopathologic Classification

Primary testicular neoplasms are divided into germinal tumors, originating from spermatogonia and their derivatives, and nongerminal tumors, which arise from Sertoli cells, epithelial cells lining the rete testis, and intersititial cells. The germinal

Table 1. The two classification systems for testicular neoplasms

Testicular Tumor Panel an Registry of Great Britain and Ireland	Armed Forces Institute of Pathology

Germinal origin
  1. Seminoma (s)
 	
Uncertain histogenesis
  1. Teratoma differentiated (TD)
  2. Malignant teratoma intermediate (MTI)
    a) MTIA — with differentiated or organoid components
    b) MTIB — no differentiated or organoid components
  3. Malignant teratoma anaplastic (MTA)
  4. Malignant teratoma trophoblastic (MTT)
 	
Combined tumor — seminoma and teratoma
 	
Sertoli cell tumor
 	
Interstitial cell tumor
 	
Orchioblastoma
 	
Others
	Germinal origin
	  1. Seminoma
	    a) Typical (classic)
	    b) Anaplastic
	    c) Spermatocytic (atypical)
	  2. Embryonal carcinoma
	  3. Teratoma
	  4. Teratoma with malignant areas (teratocarcinoma)
	  5. Choriocarcinoma
	  6. Compound tumor
	
	Nongerminal origin
	  1. Interstitial cell tumor
	  2. Gonadal-stroma tumors
	
	Miscellaneous

tumors comprise 97% of the total [23]. Currently, there are two classification systems for testicular neoplasms (Table 1). The classification of the Armed Forces Institute of Pathology is followed in the United States and throughout most of the world [99]. The other system has been proposed by the Testicular Tumor Panel and Registry of Great Britain and Ireland [19]. The two major differences between the systems are the designation of teratomas as being of uncertain histogenesis, rather than germinal origin, and rejection of the concept and use of the term embryonal carcinoma in the British classification (see Table 1). This paper will use the terminology of the Armed Forces Institute of Pathology.

Seminoma is the common histologic type of testicular cancer appearing in pure form in about 40% of cases [56] (Table 2). It is a tumor of primitive germ cells that usually are uniform and have clear cytoplasm and well-defined borders. Seminomas are subclassified into three categories: The typical or classic form, an anaplastic variety, and a spermatocytic variety; the latter is least common. Seminomas are the most common histologic type found in undescended testes. They occur in an age group about 10 years older than the other types. The testis can enlarge up to ten times its normal size and yet its normal gonadal configuration is maintained.

Table 2. Histologic breakdown of testicular tumors

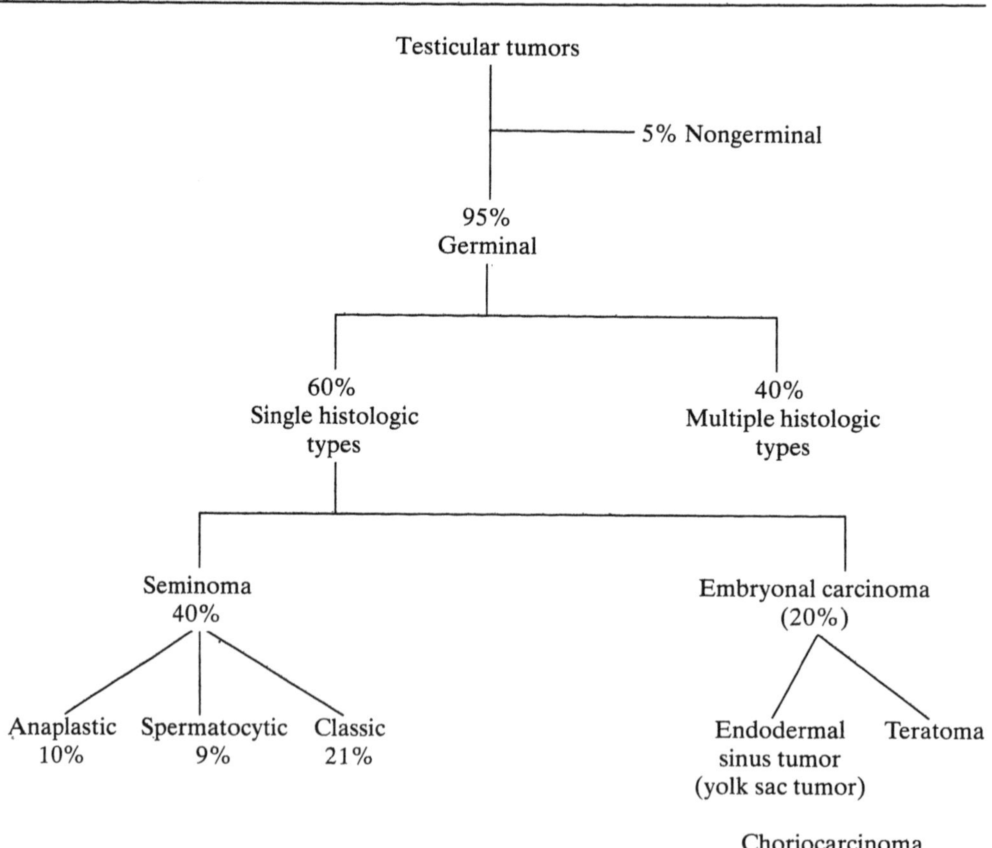

Grossly atypical, or classic seminoma, is usually smooth, homogeneous, solitary, and distinct from the surrounding parenchyma. Histologically, it is characterized by large, uniform, round or polyhedral cells resembling spermatogonia separated into lobules or cords by delicate fibrous tissue septa, containing variable numbers of mature lymphocytes and small blood vessels.

The anaplastic seminoma, is more aggressive, is generally thought to have a poorer prognosis, and accounts for about 10% of seminomas. The nuclei may be larger, more vesicular and more irregular than in typical seminoma, but increased mitotic activity is the most important and easily recognizable feature. The diagnosis is usually made where an average of three or more mitotic figures per high-power field is found. Spermatocytic seminoma occurs exclusively in the testis and has not been ssociated with teratomatous elements. It occurs most commonly over the age of 40 years and comprises 9% of seminomas. On gross examination, the tumor tends to be softer, more gelatinous, and yellow. Microscopically three different types of cells are found. The main cell type is a medium-sized cell with a round nucleus and considerable eosinophilic cytoplasm. Intermixed with these cells are small cells and giant cells, which are usually mononuclear. The tumor cells usually occur in sheets and occasionally contain lakes an eosinophilic precipate. The tumor cells have cytoplasm devoid of glycogen.

Embryonal carcinoma accounts for 15%–20% of testicular cancers. It is in most cases a much smaller tumor than seminoma. The affected testis is asymmetrically enlarged and the cut tumor surface has a gray or gray-red heterogeneous appearance. Areas of hemorrhage and necrosis are common, but gross cystic degeneration is absent. The tumor is composed of large, polygonal or oviod cells that have a primitive epithelial appearance; often they have clear cytoplasm, growing in a variety of patterns.

Teratomas are composed of mesodermal, endodermal, and ectodermal elements. The mixture of these elements varies from tumor to tumor. The great majority of teratomas are found to have well-differentiated epithelial structures lined with epithelium that is either of the keratinizing squamous type or the entero-respiratory type. These structures are usually embedded in fibromyxoid or fibrocartilaginous stroma.

Choriocarcinoma is histologically composed of cell masses of small cytotrophoblasts and large polymorphic multinucleate syncitiotrophoblasts. Admixed with the typical chorionic cells are other such as slender elongated spindle cells, and minute pyknotic cells.

Yolk sac tumors are found most commonly in children as a gonadal or sacrococcygeal neoplasm. They are composed microscopically of a network of spaces lined by small, uniform, cuboidal cells with minute cytoplasm and finely granular nuclear chromatin. The tumor cells commonly form branching cell columns or are arranged in cell nests with a central capillary vessel. These are the so-called Schiller-Duval bodies. These tumors secrete alpha-fetoprotein.

Anatomic Staging (Nonseminomatous Lesions)

Generally speaking, clinical efforts at staging have developed three broad stages as follows: Stage 1, tumor confined to the testis; stage 2, metastatic diseases in retroperitoneal lymph nodes; stage 3, metastatic lesions beyond the retroperitoneal lymph nodes. Barski [6] has advocated a modification where stage IA is a tumor confined to one testis without clinical or radiographic evidence of spread beyond

Table 3. Walter Reed Army Hospital System

Stage IA.	Tumor confined to one testis; no clinical or roentgenographic evidence of spread beyond; may include excretory or retrograde urography, lymphangiography, inferior venacavography, and chest roentgenography
Stage IB.	Same as in stage IA, but found to have histologic evidence of metastases to iliac or paraaortic lymph nodes at time of retroperitoneal lymph node dissection
Stage II.	Clinical or roentgenographic evidence of metastases to femoral, inguinal, iliac, or paraaortic lymph nodes; no demonstrable metastases above the diaphragm or to visceral organs
Stage III.	Clinical or roentgenographic evidence of metastases above the diaphragm or other distant metastases to body organs

Table 4. Royal Marsden Hospital staging system for testicular tumors

Stage I.	Confined to testis with normal lymphangiogram
Stage II.	Lymphangiography evidence of node involvement in the iliac, or paraaortic regions Evidence of spread to inguinal nodes as a result of local tumor extension or of surgical interference
Stage III.	Lymph node involvement in mediastinum or neck with or without evidence of abdominal node involvement
Stage IV.	Distant metastases

(Table 3). Stage IB is the same as stage IA with histologic evidence of metastasis to iliac or paraaortic lymph nodes at the time of lymphadnectomy. Stage II is clinical or radiographic evidence of metastasis to femoral, inguinal, iliac, or paraaortic lymph nodes with no demonstrable metastasis above the diaphragm or other distant metastasis.

In Great Britain, Boden and Ginn [12] described stages A, B, and C roughly equivalent to the U.S, stages I, II and III. Since 1962, the Royal Marsden Hospital [89] has used a four-stage classification (Table 4). The Union International Contra le Cancrum (UICC) [64] has developed a clinical stage classification (Table 5).

The American Joint Committee on Clinical Staging and End Result Reporting has essentially adapted the UICC categories with a few minor modifications [64]: (1) cT is used for preoperative clinical staging and pT is used for postoperative staging; (2) for N categories, if the finding is based on lymphangiography, 1 is inserted between N and the applicable number; (3) if histologically confirmed, + is added; if histologically negative, − is added.

A breakdown of 963 cases at Memorial Hospital staged with the TNM system is given in Table 6 [7]. In the Memorial Hospital series there was a reasonable correlation of clinical and pathological staging (Table 7). The staging breakdown could be significantly related to histology. Distant metastases at the time of initial diagnosis were most common in choriocarcinoma (80%) and rarest in pure seminoma (4%) (Table 8). The corallary was that the highest incidence of patients presenting with

Table 5. UICC clinical stage classification of testicular tumors

T	
T1	Tumor limited to body of testis
T2	Tumor extending beyond tunica
T3	Tumor involving rete testis or epididymis
T4	Tumor invading spermatic cord
T4a	Tumor invading spermatic cord
T4b	Tumor invading scrotal wall
N	Regional = Paraaortic, paracaval and homolateral inguinal nodes
	Juxtaregional = Intrapelvic, mediastinal and supraclavicular nodes
N1	Single homolateral regional node involvement
N2	Contralateral or bilateral multiple regional nodes
N3	Palpable abdominal mass or fixed inguinal nodes
N4	Involvement of juxtaregional nodes
M	
M1	Distant metastases
M1a	Evidence of occult metastases based on biochemical and/or other tests
M1b	Single metastasis in a single organ site
M1c	Multiple metastasis in a single organ site
M1d	Metastasis in multiple organ sites)

Table 6. TNM staging of testicular cancer in 963 patients at Memorial Hospital [7]

T	Number
1 Confined to testis proper	891
2 Involvement of tunica albuginea	8
3 Involvement of rete testis of epididymis	20
4 Involvement of spermatic cord	44
N (with m_0)	
0 Nodes uninvolved	475
1 Involvement of cord nodes	22
2 Involvement of multiple nodes	205
3 With palpable abdominal mass	26
4 Juxtaregional lymphatic metastases	72
M_1	163
(N_0–N_4)	

Table 7. Correlation of clinical and pathologic staging in testicular carcinoma at Memorial Hospital 1949–1974 [7].

Number clinically staged	424	
Number pathologic stage same	328	(77%)
Number pathologic stage ↑	87	(21%)
Number pathologic stage ↓	9	(2%)

Table 8. Distant metastases at the time of initial diagnosis at Memorial Hospital 1949–1974, 963 cases [7]

	%
Pure seminoma	4
Teratocarcinoma	15
Embryonal carcinoma	17
Choriocarcinoma	80

Table 9. Percentage of patients with testicular cancer presenting N_0M_0 at Memorial Hospital 1949–1974 [7], 963 cases

	%
Pure seminoma	75
Teratocarcinoma	50
Embryonal	27
Pure choriocarcinoma	10

Table 10. Clinical staging of testicular carcinoma

History
Physical Examination
CBC, urine
Liver chemistries
BUN, creatinine
Chest X-ray
Whole lung tomography
IVP
Bipedal lymphangiogram
Retroperitoneal CAT scans and/or ultrasound
Quantitative pre- and post-orchiectomy serum radioimmunoassay of HCG and AFP

NoMo lesions was in pure seminoma (75%), while it was lowest in pure choriocarcinoma (10%) (Table 9).

The clinical staging for the evaluation of possible extrogonadal matastatic disease after orchiectomy usually includes a variety of tests (Table 10).

After routine posterior-anterior and lateral chest radiographs have been performed to look for pulmonary metastases, full lung tomograms will identify an additional 3%–6% of patients with pulmonary metastases when none were observed on plain films [25]. When computerized tomography (CT) scans are used, the sensitivity but not the specificity in finding lung metastases is increased [84].

The scalene lymph nodes may be the first site of extraabdominal tumor. This can occur as tumor cells may move through the thoracic duct. Donohue et al [24] routinely biopsied scalene nodes in 57 patients and found additional disease in five (9%). One or more of these scalene lymph nodes are frequently opacified by pedal lymphangiograms as the first site of extraabdominal metastatic spread.

Recently, Lynch and Richie [52] have reported that supraclavicular node biopsies in 73 patients with testis tumors revealed tumor in only four patients; this broke down to 3/61 patients with nonseminomatous lesions and 1/12 with seminoma. All four of the positive patients on biopsy were known to have other metastases and in three of the four a palpable supraclavicular mass was noted as well. The low yield of the procedure combined with an 8% complication rate leads the authors to recommend against the routine use of supraclavicular node biposy in patients without a supraclavicular mass.

Buck et al. [14] reported on 38 consecutive patients who underwent supraclavicular node biopsy as a part of the initial evaluation. As part of their preoperative studies, they all had a bilateral pedal lymphangiogram and an inferior vena cavagram. Technically satisfactory visualization of the supraclavicular nodes after lymphangiography was achieved in 24 patients. In eight patients the thoracic duct was visualized but not the nodes, and in six neither was seen. There were 15 stage I patients (Walter-Reed classification) and 23 who stage II. Three patients had histologically documented metastatic tumor in the supraclavicular nodes. All of these had stage II disease. Two falsely positive diagnoses were made prior to biopsy. In both cases all that was found was lipogranulomatous lymphadenitis.

This series indicated that supraclavicular node biopsy was most helpful in evaluating patients with unequivocally positive abdominal lymphangiograms and negative chest X-rays. Of this group (clinically, stage II), 13% were found to be stage III with this procedure. This series was reported prior to the use of markers and one wonders if these three patients found to be positive on supraclavicular node biopsy would have been found to have elevated markers, which would have obviated the need.

An inferior vena cavagraphy (IVP) is an essential aspect of staging since it can detect ureteral obstruction and occasionally renal vein obstruction. Appropriate prompt therapy may save a kidney threatened by ureteral obstruction. Inferior vena cavagraphy with or without selective renal vein injections may give evidence of additional intraabdominal metastases not seen by lymphangiography [51]. This results from total replacement of a lymph node preventing opacification by ethiodol, or by metastases to lymph nodes that are not normally opacified, such as the renal hilum or above the systerna chili.

One of the major problems encountered in all clinical staging systems is the inability to diagnose fully intraabdominal lymph node involvement without surgical exploration. Pedal lymphangiography closes this gap to a significant degree. Wallace and Jing [108] have reported that both surgical and autopsy findings correlated with the results observed in pedal lymphangiograms. Of 18 cases with a positive roentgenographic interpretation, 17 (94) had a positive finding in the nodes at surgical exploration. In 49 negative lymphangiograms, only eight proved to be false negative after lymphadenectomy.

The testicular lymphatics follow the testicular veins such that left-sided tumors tend to metastasize to the left renal hilum and high left paraaortic lymph nodes at approximately the L_2 level. Tumors on the right side tend to drain directly into the right paraaortic and paracaval lymph nodes at the L_2L_3 level, slightly lower than those on the left. Alternate lymphatic pathways are occasionally seen, such as metastasis from testicular tumors to the parailiac or inguinal nodes. When tumors have extended outside the testis, other lymphatic spraed pathways have been observed.

The technique of lymphangiography involves cannulation of a lymphatic vessel in the foot and the injection of ethiodol. This is followed by anterio posterior (AP) views of the abdomen, pelvis and thoracic duct. The next day, AP, oblique and lateral X-rays of the abdomen and pelvis are taken as well as a PA of the chest. In the region of a primary metastatic involvement, it is important to note any disorganization or displacement of the lymphatic vessels. Those vessels involved with the tumor may terminate abruptly and evidence of collateral circulation may be seen. Possible obstruction of lymphatic vessels is indicated by residual contrast material in lymphatic vessels or delayed films 24 h later. Gross collateral circulation points toward an interpretation of profound replacemant of the nodes by metastasis.

Nodal involvement will result in a node appearing enlarged in all dimensions. Large filling defects measuring 5 mm or more should be regarded as suspicious. The differential diagnosis must involve granulomatous disease, lipomatosis, and follicles. Nodes with large metastatic deposits may show the crescent or flare sign in which the nodal tissue is compressed so that a thin crescentric rim is visualized. A completely replaced node will not be visualized and so will be missed by this technique.

Depending upon which side the primary lesion has been found, different patterns of nodal involvement have been described. With right-sides lesions, metastatic involvement is seen predominately in the paracaval nodes at the level of L2−3, together with involvement of the interaortocava group of nodes and, more rarely, the left upper paraaortic nodes when the disease is extensive. With primary lesions on the left side, the nodes involved commonly are those in the upper para- and preaortic region, relating to the junction of the testicular vein and the left regional vein. The aortocaval nodes will be involved when obstruction of para- and preaortic nodes has occurred. Involvement of the entire left paraaortic chain is occasionally seen after obstruction to the primary center with retrograde involement of nodes by metastates.

Lymphangiograms in testicular tumors have an overall accuracy of about 85%. The specificity is 80% (with a 20% false-negative rate), while the sensitivity is in the 90% range. The high false-negative rate is caused by micrometastases too small to be visualized by this technique and is also caused by the failure to render nodes totally replaced by tumor paque.

Computerized tomography provides another dimension in visualizing the retroperitoneum. It can identify both paraaortic and parailiac lymph nodes. In addition, masses can also be observed in regions that are otherwise difficult to visualize such as the renal and splenic hila and retrocrural areas. Ancillary information such as the detection of hepatic metastases may also be gained.

Computerized tomography can detect differences as small as 0.1% in the attenuation of X-ray photons by adjacent tissues to produce a cross-sectional image. Fat provides a low-density contrast medium, which can neatly outline internal structures. Because of this, patients, especially those with depleted fat due to chronic cancer, are the most difficult to evaluate.

Burney and Klatte [15] have reviewed their experience with 290 ultrasound examinations and 188 CT examinations in 136 testicular cancer patients with prior orchiectomies. The examinations were reinterpreted and the results compared with the original reports and the clinical, surgical, and pathologic findings.

Reininterpretation results agreed with the first report in 83% of examinations for ultrasound and 87% of computerized axial tomography (CAT) scans. Interobserver agreement was 80% for ultrasound and 88% for CT. The accuracy for retroperitoneal lymphadnectomy for the two approaches was as follows:

Ultrasound	Computerized tomography
7% false positive	7% false positive
15% false negative	12% false negative
72% correct	73% correct
7% equivocal	6% equivocal

When ultrasound and CAT scans were performed on the same patient within 1 week of one another and interpreted as if they represent a single examination the interobserver agreement was 92%. The accuracy analysis shows 0% false positive, 14% false negative, 74% correct, and 12% equivocal.

Tumor Markers

Alpha-fetoprotein (AFP) is a protein with a molecular weight of 70,000 synthesized by the parenchymal cells of the liver, yolk sac, and gastrointestinal tract of the fetus [1, 34, 66]. At 12–15 weeks of gestation, levels as high as 3,000,000 ng/ml have been measured [107]. The levels fall to 10,000–150,000 ng/ml at birth and at 1 year of age AFP is usually not detectable by immunoprecipitation methods. Recently, radioimmunoassays and enzyme immunoassays have been developed that can detect the 1–16 ng/ml levels present in normal serum. Extensive studies on normal controls have established 40 ng/ml or above as a clearly abnormal level. Waldmann and McIntyre [107] reported that 75 of 101 patients with nonseminomatous testicular germ cell tumors of all stages had elevated AFP levels.
Human chorionic gonadotropin (HCG) is a hormone secreted by the syncytiotrophoplastic cells of the normal placenta. Serum elevations are observed in nearly all patients with gestational trophoblastic disease. It is a glycoprotein with a molecular weight of 45,000 containing two dissimilar polypeptide units designated alpha and beta. Vaitukaitus et al. [102] have developed a radioimmunoassay for the hormone using antibodies to the beta chain. Normal serum levels are below 1 ng/ml. Scardino et al. [83] have reported that 73 of 100 patients with testicular nonseminomatous germ cell tumors had an elevated HCG level.
When both potential markers were looked at together by the National Cancer Institute, in their initial study, 50 of the first 100 patients had an elevation of both AFP and HCG. In addition, 16 had an elevated of AFP alone and 14 of HCG alone. Only 11 patients had neither marker elevated.
In a prospective study [43], none of the 55 patients had an elevation of the markers when a benign testicular mass was confirmed after orchiectomy. On the other hand, 11 of 14 patients with a malignant mass had marker elevation. Thus, there were no false-positive values for these markers but there was a false-negative rate of 21%. Therefore, in diagnosis of a scrotal mass, the markers cannot be used as the basis for a therapeutic decision.
In a prospective study to evaluate the accuracy of markers in the staging work-up, again the value was adjunctive but not definitive. Scardino et al [83] studied 31 clinically stage I patients. Eleven subsequently were shown to have tumor involvement in the retroperitoneal nodes at lymphadnectomy. Six of these patients had an elevation

of one or both markers postorchiectomy, which correctly indicated the presence of occult metastases. The staging discrepancy was therefore reduced from 35% (11 of 31), based on clinical and lymphangiogram data alone, to 16% (5 of 31), based on the additional information provided by the markers. In this study, six patients were clinically stage II; only four had elevated markers while the remaining two, with negative nodes, had normal marker levels. Therefore, the discrepancy in clinical staging in these six patients was reduced from 33% (two of six), based on clinical data, to 0% Cnone of six), based on the marker level.

The value of determining marker levels prior to retroperitoneal lymphadnectomy must take cognizance of the metabolic clearance of the two markers. This is more true for AFP with its longer half-line than it is for HCG. A single elevated marker just before or after lymphadnectomy cannot be used to determine the presence of metastases because it could reflect either the continued presence of tumor or a normally falling serum titer after removal of all marker-producing neoplasm. What is needed is at least two values taken several days apart so that one can calculate the expected value by constructing a curve.

When all factors of metabolic decay are accounted for, the false-negative rate prior to lymphadnectomy will be in the range of 20%–40%. These are predominantly in patients with microscopic nodal metastases. What still needs to be fully determined is what is the most cost-effective mix of lymphangiograms, CAT scans, ultrasound, and markers in clinical staging after orchiectomy. Both Lange et al. [17] and Scardino et al [83] report that markers diminish staging errors by 10%–25%. Marker determination cannot be used in lieu of other staging procedures because there are instances when the marker levels are normal while the other diagnostic modalities correctly diagnose retroperitoneal metastasis. The general consensus at this time is that markers cannot be used safely to avoid a lymphadnectomy.

The major values for marker determinations prior to lymphadnectomy are as follows: (1) If the preoperative and immediately postoperative values are known, one may diagnose unappreciated persistent disease earlier. This will have great relevance in decision making about further adjuvant therapy. (2) Some patients are serologically stage II only. That is, prelymphadnectomy marker levels are truly elevated but no disease is found in the lymph nodes on pathologic examination. After surgery, the marker levels fall according to metabolic decay rates thereby confirming that marker-producing tumor was removed. These cases may fall into a separate prognostic group. (3) A knowledge of whether a tumor does or does not produce elevated serum marker levels may have prognostic significance. (4) Advances in staging techniques and new or more sensitive tumor markers may increase the possibility that noninvasive methods of staging will ultimately prove reliable. This will be facilitated by continued prospective marker determinations.

The greatest value of marker determinations is in serial monitoring after surgery for stage I and II disease and after chemotherapy for advanced disease. Lange et al [17] have followed 173 patients with nonseminomatous testicular cancers with marker studies from the time of initial active disease for as long as 35 months. They found that the marker value usually reflects or predicts the progression or remission of disease with a lead time of as long as 6 months. There were no false positive in patients known or later confirmed to be free of disease. The false-negative rate in 125 stage III patients was 10%. These false-negative were of several types: (1) Patients were consistently negative from the onset of disease; (2) the patients were marker-positive at diagnosis but were negative at the time of tumor recurrence or persistently active disease; (3) the patients elevated markers declined to normal, yet clinical evidence of disease regressed more slowly and eventually disappeared as chemotherapy continued. Marker elevations are being observed in seminomas. The exact incidence of HCG is probably in the range of 5%−10%. When AFP is elevated, this is irrefutable evidence for the existence of nonseminomatous testicular neoplasm being present and the patients should be treated accordingly even without pathologic documentation. When only HCG is found elevated, radiation can still be used but every attempt should be made to prove the tumor to be pure seminoma.

Kohn [45] from England has also warned that the return of AFP levels toward normal in testicular teratoma is not necessarily indicative of a cure. It is the half-life that is critical to the determination. The natural AFP $\tau_{1/2}$ is 4−6 days which is what will be observed if all tumor tissue has been eradicated. A slower rate of decline and persistence of AFP correlates well with residual tumor. The development of an abnormally apparent half-life ($\tau_{1/2}$ modified by continued tumor production) may be the first indication of treatment failure preceding a rise in AFP and clinical tumor recurrence. Kohn recommends that to monitor treatment response, serum sampling should start at twice a week and then proceed to weekly for 4−6 weeks.

Therapeutic Implications of Staging

In testicular cancer, pathologic staging plays an important role as does clinical staging but the therapeutic implications are not a dominating factor. Orchiectomy in all cases is performed for diagnostic purposes and staging within the tumor compartment carries little therapeutic implications and not a great deal of prognostic implications. Regardless of the extent of tumor spread within the primary organ, additional therapy addressing the problem of regional lymph node control should be undertaken unless clinical staging determines that metastasis exist. Clinical staging with lymphangiography, while of prognostic value, will in most cases not changes a planned secondary therapeutic attack with either surgery or X-rays. If lymphadnectomy is performed, pathologic staging can be precisely determined with important prognostic implications for metastatic relapse. The only immediate therapeutic implication would relate to the use of adjuvant systemic treatment.

Therapeutic Approaches

Surgery, radiotherapy, and chemotherapy have all been useful in patients with testicular tumors and immunotherapy may ultimately play an important therapeutic role. The problem facing clinicians is how to combine these modalities into optimum programs of therapy.

Surgery

Surgery finds application in the treatment of the primary tumor and regional lymphatic metastases, and in the management of distant metastases. Surgical removal of the primary tumor is always indicated immediately after the clinical diagnosis. This also permits serial section of the testis to determine the proper histopathologic diagnosis.

Table 11. Results of primary treatment with lymphadnectomy and postoperative radiotherapy

Investigator	Stage I			Stage II		
	No. of patients	No. NED 3–5 years	% NED	No. of patients	No. NED 3–5 years	% NED
Whitmore [114]	204	184	90	159	78	49
Walsh et al. [109]	44	41	93	20	12	60
Bradfield et al. [13]	40	28	70	34	11	32
Skinner [87]	30	27	90	27	15	56
Maier and Sulak [56]	109	80	73	97	44	45
Staubitz et al. [95]	17	15	88	8	7	88

The current practice is to perform an orchiectomy that includes high inguinal ligation of the vas and spermatic vessels, complete removal of the contents of the inguinal canal, and removal of the testis and its adnexa, including the parietal layer of the tunica vaginalis.

Any time a scrotal mass is found in which any suspicion of a testis tumor exists, an inguinally approached orchiectomy is mandatory. The inguinal cord is clamped and preferably divided before the tunics are stretched and the testis expressed into the wound. This prior clamping prevents tumor emboli via the cord. It is important that the patient understand preoperatively that loss of one testicle will not impair sexual function or fertility. The patient should understand that one testis is expendable and that the operation is not a biopsy or an exploration.

After orchiectomy, all the slides must be reviewed by an experienced pathologist. This can lead to an altered diagnosis in the type of germinal cell testicular tumor in approximately 20% of patients referred. This is understandable given the relative infrequency in which a general pathologist in a community hospital is called upon to diagnose these uncommon tumors. The important discrimination by the pathologist is pure seminoma vs nonseminomatous malignant lesions.

There is undoubtedly a curative potential in orchiectomy alone but it is rarely, if ever, used as the sole treatment [113]. Since the prime mechanism of metastasis is by the lymphatics and the retroperitoneal lymph nodes are the usual initial sites of dissemination, all clinical groups treat these nodes in some manner. Experience in the last 25 years has shown that surgery to remove the primary lymphatic drainage may be accomplished with a low mortality and acceptable morbidity. In the series of Whitmore [112] and Staubitz et al. [96], combined orchiectomy and retroperitoneal lymph node dissection produced a 5-year survival rate of 87% in patients with 'negative' lymph nodes irrespective of tumor type. In the cases of 'positive' nodes, the survival rate was 66%. A summary of surgical results in stage I and II disease is given in Table 11.

Radiotherapy

Radiotherapy is appropriate in the management of both retroperitoneal lymph node metastases and distant metastases, and may be either curative or palliative depending

Table 12. Results of primary treatment with radiotherapy following orchiectomy

Investigator	Stage I			Stage II		
	No. of patients	No. NED 3–5 years	% NED	No. of patients	No. NED 3–5 years	% NED
Van Derwerf-Messing [103]	29	26	90	35	16	40
Peckham and McElwain [71]	78	66	85	29	17	59
Batterman et al. [8]	30	21	70	19	5	26
Maier and Mittemayer [55]	29	25	86	11	9	82
	166	138	83	94	47	50

upon the circumstances. Irradiation may be used to destroy metastatic foci in the lymph nodes without producing clinically important damage to adjacent normal tissues. Radiotherapy has a technical advantage over surgery in that there are no skipped areas at the target end of a properly directed beam.

The results of the primary treatment of nonseminomatous stage I and II lesions with radiotherapy following orchiectomy is outlined in Table 12 from four major series.

The Local Control Dilemma

For the nonseminomatous types, which are often lumped together as 'carcinoma', the controversy over apparent local control is great. After orchiectomy and clinical staging, the options include (1) surgery only, (2) radiotherapy only, (3) radiotherapy – surgery – radiotherapy, (4) chemotherapy or any additional combinations that could be devised. There exist no controlled clinical trial data that prove the value of one approach more than another.

Regardless of the therapeutic option utilized, stage I disease is highly curable. A cure-rate of 85% will be achieved by orchiectomy followed by lymphadnectomy alone, irradiation alone, or the two together (Table 13). At Memorial Hospital, an adjuvant chemotherapy program of actinomycin ± chlorambucil for 2 years did not improve on this result [114]. Skinner [87] has compared his retrospective experience in both stage I and II treated with adjuvant drug versus no treatment and found a survival rate of 93% in the former and 82% in the latter.

At Stanford [26], a so-called sandwich technique patients with stage I and II carcinoma (clinical staging) was evaluated and the patients were initially given 3,000 rad to the abdominal lymph nodes. This was followed by a 3-week rest period at the end of which each patient was evaluated by an abdominal roentgenogram to study dye-filled lymph nodes and full-lung tomography to search for pulmonary metastases. A bilateral retroperitoneal lymph nodes dissection was then performed; radiation therapy was resumed.

Table 13. 5-year survival in stage I nonseminatous testicular cancer

Author	Treatment	No. treated	No. disease free at 5 years	%
Whitmore [114]	Orchiectomy and lymphadnectomy	49	43	86
Boctor et al. [11]	Orchiectomy and lymphadnectomy	13	8	62
Walsh et al. [109]	Orchiectomy and lymphadnectomy	35	24	69
Staubitz et al. [95]	Orchiectomy and lymphadnectomy	36	31	86
Walsh et al. [109]	Orchiectomy lymphadnectomy and postoperative irradiation	19	17	89
Maier and Mittemayer [55]	Orchiectomy lymphadnectomy and postoperative irradiation	162	120	70
Peckham and McElwain [71]	Orchiectomy and irradiation	63	54	86

Initially, the ports were the same as those used preoperatively. However, oblique fields were employed to deliver over 4,000 rad to the periaortic lymph nodes. The total dose was usually 4,000 rad to the periaortic lymph nodes. The total dose was usually 5,000 rad when the dissection was negative and 5,500 rad when positive. When the abdominal lymph nodes were involved, 4,500–5,000 rad were given to the mediastinum and supraclavicular regions.

At Stanford, a retrospective comparison with the standard radiotherapy approach has shown no definite value for the sandwich technique except that it allows the separation of patients who do very well from those who will do less well.

Maier and Mittemeyer [55] have reported a prospective randomized study comparing radiation alone with the 'sandwich technique' (pre- and postlymphadnectomy radiation) for stage I and II disease. The disease-free survival at 3 years was not significantly different for the two approaches in stage I patients. With irradiation alone it was 86% (25/29), while for the combined approach it was 97% (29/30). In stage II, the radiation alone was 82% (9/11) as compared to 81% (17/21) for the 'sandwich' approach. These results demonstrate that radiotherapy can achieve as high a percentage of long-term surviving as has been reported previously for lymphadnectomy alone. Combining the two modalities appears to offer no survival advantage.

Stage II testicular carcinoma is the stage where all of the therapeutic modalities converge. The possibilities for interaction between the three modalities in stage II are numerous, yet the available clinical trial patient resources are uncommon. For each modality there are critical questions which need to be asked to firmly establish the comparative cost-benefit ratios for their application.

The options for stage II disease after orchiectomy become quite numerous (Table 14). The relative roles for radiation vs surgery have not been clearly established at this

Table 14. A perspective on adjuvant chemotherapy of testicular cancer. Ten possibilities for treatment of stage II nonseminomatous testicular carcinoma

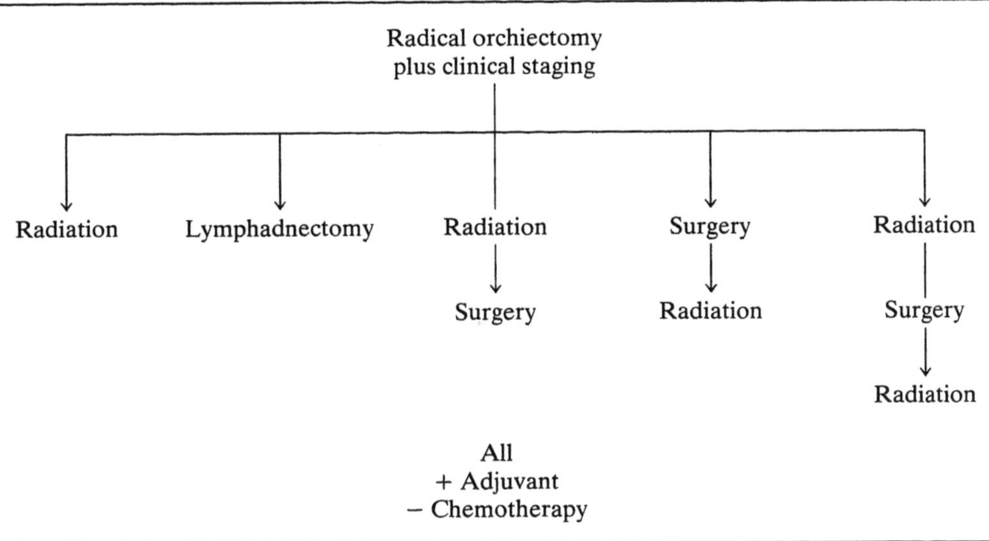

time. Both modalities alone have been reported to give roughly comparable results in noncomparable retrospective literature reports. The lack of comparability in these reports involves differences in case selection, clinical staging, as well as data reporting techniques involving aspects such as exclusions.

One of the problems in comparing testicular cancer treated with lymphadnectomy or radiation only is that surgical staging is precise, as compared to clinical staging in the radiation groups. After lymphadnectomy, a subgroup of patients with microscopic involvement of the nodes would be placed in the stage II category. In radiation-treated groups these patients would still be called stage I. This would tend to bias results in favor of surgery and radiation oncologists have argued that the comparability of results between the two modalities for 'stage I' disease is, therefore, a possible evidence of the superiority of radiation.

When the 3 year relapse-free survival rate in stage II for the three major approaches are compared, little difference can be seen although the numbers are quite small.

Seminomas

Seminoma is clearly the most radiosensitive and radiocurable tumor. Friedman [33] has found that the lethal dose for seminoma is in the range of 1,000 rad in 10−14 days. By comparison, the dose for 'carcinoma' is 4,000−5,000 rad in 3−6 weeks, although an occasional tumor may be atypically sensitive to a lethal dose of 2,500−3,000 rad in 2−3 weeks. Seminomas have their own staging system (Table 15). Since the seminomas are highly radiosensitive, therapy for stage I lesions is orchiectomy and irradiation. Stage I is defined as a negative lymphangiogram and/or low abdominal ultrasound and CT. Since lymphadnectomy is not routinely performed, the exact percentage of stage I

Table 15. Testicular seminoma staging system

Stage I.	Tumor limited to the testicle with no evidence of spread through the capsule or to the cord
Stage II.	Evidence of tumor extending beyond the testicle but not beyond the regional lymphatic drainage, including patients with tumor in the spermatic cord, scrotum, inguinal, iliac, or periaortic nodes
Stage III.	Involvement beyond the diaphragma, but confined to the lymphatic system or massive retroperitoneal disease
Stage IV.	Generalized abdominal, visceral, bone, pulmonary, or other distant metastases

patients who actually have involvement of the retroperitoneal nodes is unknown. The cure rate for stage I lesions with irradiation after orchiectomy is 95%−100%.

Stage II disease is defined as a positive lymphangiogram and palpable abdominal mass with no evidence of metastases. The treatment is still irradiation with a cure rate of 75%−90% to be expected. Prophylactic irradiation to the mediastinum and left supraclavicular fossa is routinely added to abdominal radiotherapy for patients with stage II disease.

Stage III seminoma is defined as lymphatic involvement above the diaphragm involving cervical and/or mediastinal nodes. This stage accounts for only 5% of seminomas, so large series are not available. Einhorn and Williams [31] recommend that these patients should be treated initially with combination chemotherapy and consolidated with X-ray therapy if needed. This recommendation would be particularly true in anaplastic seminomas in this stage, where radiotherapy alone has practically no cure potential.

The Memorial Hospital group has attempted to analyze their seminoma experience utilizing a TNM staging approach, and their 5-year survival results are given in Table 16.

Percarpio et al. [73] have reviewed the extensive Walter-Reed Army Hospital experience with anaplastic seminomas over a 28-year period beginning in 1950. In this period, 82 patients were diagnosed as having anaplastic seminoma out of a total of 405 patients with pure seminoma of all three subtypes for a frequency of 20%. Of these, 58 patients presented with stage I disease and 19 with stage II disease. Five patients presented with stage III disease.

The median age of the patients was 30 years at diagnosis with a range of 18−53 years. Of these men, 13% developed their neoplasm in an undescended testis or in a testis that had undergone orchiopexy. The median follow-up time in this analysis was 97 months.

The stage I patients received doses of 2,000−2,500 rad to the paraaortic, ipsilateral pelvic, and inguinal lymph nodes. Of the 58 patients so treated, two have died of their seminoma after developing diffuse metastases outside their irradiated fields at 9 and 16 months after diagnosis. The 5- and 10-year actuarial survival rates for stage I patients are 96%. Of the 58 patients with stage I lesions, 35 also received mediastinal and supraclavicular irradiation in addition to subdiaphragmatic treatment. The results in this group are in no way superior to these of the 23 patients who received abdominal irradiation only.

Table 16. 5-year survival for 304 seminomas treated at Memorial Hospital (1949–1974) correlated with TNM staging

	No. of patients	No. alive 5 years	%
Local			
N_0M_0	227	200	88
Regional			
N_1	0	0	0
N_2			
Microscopic	2	2	100
Gross	37	24	65
N_3			
Palpable	8	4	50
N_4	19	10	53
Pelvic	6	3	50
Inguinal	3	2	67
Mediastinal	10	5	50
Supraclavicular			
Distant			
$N_0-N_4\ m_1$	11	3	27
	304	243	80

The 5- and 10-year survival rates for the 28 stage II patients are 87% in this series. Two patients died with widespread lung and visceral metastases at 23 and 29 months following diagnosis. Therefore, a total of four patients with stage I and II disease developed widespread metastasis. In all four patients the metastases were also anaplastic seminoma in biopsy confirmed in three of then at autopsy. No patients developed metastases of a nonseminomatous variety.

Early in this series, 14 patients had lymphadnectomy in addition to irradiation. These were 12 patients with stage I and 2 with stage II. Four of these patients developed gastrointestinal complications requiring laparotomy. In contrast, only 1 of 63 patients treated with irradiation developed treatment-related gastrointestinal complications.

In 78 patients tested HCG elevation was found in only four. Two of these patients had elevated urinary HCG titers prior to therapy (stage I) and have had prolonged disease-free survival. Two other patients had elevated serum beta-subunit titers prior to therapy (both stage II) and both expired with recurrent malignancy.

Chemotherapy

Chemotherapeutic agents have been used in the treatment of primary tumor and regional lymphatic metastases, and in managing distant metastatic disease. Adjuvant chemotherapy is also finding an increasing role in the management of patients with all stages of disease.

Table 17. Alkylating agent therapy of testicular tumors

Drug (reference)	Dose schedule	No evaluable patients	No responses[a]		Response rate	
			CR	PR	CR	CR +PR
Phenylalanine mustard [17]	50 mg 30 or 20 mg/week, PO to a total dose of 200–250 mg per course	86	–	49	–	57%
Chlorambucil [54]	10 mg/day, PO as tolerated	8	2	2	25%	50%
Cyclophosphamide [90]	8 mg/kg/day × 6 IV (case 1) 4 mg/kg/day × 60 PO (case 2)	2[b]	2	–	100%	100%

[a] *CR*, complete response; *PR*, partial response
[b] Both seminomas

Single Agents

When one evaluates the available data for chemotherapy of testicular neoplasms, a reversal of the usual approach to the chemotherapy of solid tumors is readily apparent because the data for drug combinations are more extensive than that for single agents. The combination data do not evolve from single-agent information but begin almost parallel with it.

Table 17 summarizes the data for single alkylating agents. Only phenylalanine mustard appears to have been extensively evaluated and most of the information is from the Soviet Union. Chebotareva [17] has reported 86 patients with advanced testicular tumors treated once weekly with gradually decreasing oral doses. Of 42 patients with seminomas, 38 (90%) had objective responses and 19 of these were "alive and fit for work" 2–6 years after the initiation of treatment. All but two of these patients were admitted with stage IV disease. Responses were also noted in 11 of 16 'teratoseminomas' (embryonal cell carcinoma?) but none were observed in 28 cases of chorionepithelioma. Chebotareva noted that the primary tumor generally appeared less sensitive to chemotherapy than did its metastases.

Mackenzie et al. [54] treated eight patients with chlorambucil at a dose of 10 mg daily for 13–66 days per course. Four seminoma patients responded, two by complete regression, but no response was seen in the other four patients. One of the complete responders died of the disease after 19 months but the other was living and well after over 20 months. The authors felt that chlorambucil alone could be recommended as the chemotherapy of choice for seminoma.

The data for cyclophosphamide are restricted to a report of complete regression in two cases of seminoma [90].

Very little information is available on the efficacy of the antimetabolite class of drugs (Table 18). Wyatt and McAninch [119] used methotrexate alone in ten patients with metastatic embryonal cell carcinoma, administering 2.5–5.0 mg/day PO as tolerated in as nearly continuous a fashion as possible. They reported 'spectacular tumor regression' in four patients who survived for more than 5 years. The other six patients did not respond and their mean survival was 4 months. The chief toxic effects were

Table 18. Antimetabolite therapy of testicular tumors

Drug (reference)[b]	Dose schedule	No evaluable patients	No responses[a]		Response rate	
			CR	PR	CR	CR +PR
Methotrexate [119]	2.5−5 mg/day PO to toxicity	10	−	4	−	40%
5-FU [118]	Standard loading dose (SLD)	3	−	1	−	33%
5 FU [2]	SLD	3	−	1	−	33%
5 FU [39]	SLD	4	−	1	−	25%

[a] *CR*, complete response; *PR*, partial response
[b] 5-FU − total response 3/10 = 30%

Table 19. Vinca alkaloid therapy of testicular tumors

Drug (reference)[b]	Dose schedule	No evaluable patients	No responses[a]		Response rate	
			CR	PR	CR	CR +PR
Vincristine [20]	Weekly	2	−	1	−	50%
Vincristine [110]	40 2× weekly × 2 doses, then 2−3 mg/week	2	−	1	−	50%
Vincristine [85]	50−75 kg/week IV	3	−	2	−	66%
Vinblastine [79]	0.4−0.8 mg/kg/week	21	4	7	19%	52%
Vinblastine [88]	0.1−0.3 mg/kg/week	4	−	2	−	50%

[a] *CR*, complete response; PR, partial response
[b] Vincristine total response 4/7 (57%)
   Vinblastine total response 13/25 (52%)

leukopenia and stomatitis. There were no deaths but two patients had life-threatening episodes of sepsis associated with myelosuppression.

Apparently, 5-fluorouracil has demonstrated activity against testicular tumors in a few patients included in three broad studies [2, 39, 118]. No data are available for 6-mercaptopurine, 6-thioguanine, of cytosine arabinoside. Hydroxyurea, which is a cell-cycle-specific agent although not an antimetaboite, has exhibited some activity with two responses seen among six patients treated with 40 mg/kg/day; one of these was a complete regression in an embryonal carcinoma [79].

Table 19 includes the results obtained with vinca alkaloids. Vincristine has shown a hint of activity in three broad phase II studies [20, 85, 110] that included seven patients having testicular neoplasms; overall response rate was 57% (4/7). Vinblastine has been studied to a somewhat greater extent. Samuels and Howe [79] used the drug quite intensively (0.4−0.8 mg/kg/week) and reported four complete and seven partial responses among a variety of cell types in 21 patients. Smart et àl. [88] administered a more standard dosage and obtained two partial responses.

Table 20. Mithramycin therapy of testicular tumors

Reference[b]	Dose schedule	No evaluable patients	No responses[a]		Response rate	
			CR	PR	CR	CR +PR
54	25–50 γ/kg/day × 3–10	8	–	3	–	37%
75	Various but mostly 25–50 γ/kg/day × 7–10 IV	305	33	80	10%	37%
76	25 γ/kg/day × 9–10 constant IV infusion	26	2	7	7%	35%
120	Daily and EOD	52	15	10	29%	48%

[a] *CR*, complete response; *PR*, partial response
[b] The data of Pitts [75] may include some of that in the rest of the table so overall results are not totaled

Table 21. Mithramycin in testicular tumors breakdown of response by cell type [75]

Testicular tumor type	Total	Complete response	Partial response	% response
Embryonal cell	173	26	42	40
Teratoma	5	0	1	20
Teratocarcinoma	23	0	5	21
Seminoma	18	0	7	40
Choriocarcinoma	13	1	6	53
Mixed tumor	73	6	19	34
	305	33	80	37

The antitumor antibiotics, particularly mithramycin, have been by far the most extensively studied of all the single chemotherapeutic agents (Table 20). The data compiled by Pitts [75] showed a complete response rate of 10% (33/3095) and a 27% (80/305) partial response rate for an overall response of 37% (113/305). Responses were noted in all cell types but the embryonal cell lesions were apparently the most sensitive, particularly when complete regression was viewed selectively (Table 21). Evaluation of the relationship between prior therapy and the effectiveness of mithramycin (Table 22) revealed no appreciable effect on response rate, except possibly in cases of previous treatment with actinomycin D.

Unfortunately, the number of patients evaluated was quite small and the question of clinic cross-resistance between mithramycin and actinomycin D is a crucial one that remains to be answered.

Mithramycin is not an innocuous drug and the Pfizer Company has evaluated its toxic side effects in 900 cancer patients. The most common toxic reaction was nausea and vomiting in 40%–45% of patients; interestingly, the incidence of diarrhea and stomatitis was only 1% and 2%, respectively. The hematologic abnormalities included

Table 22. Relationship of prior therapy to mithramycin response [75]

Type of prior therapy	Number patients	Response to mithramycin	No. response to mithramycin
Combination of methotrexate, chlorambucil, actinomycin D	41	16 (39.0%)	25 (61.0%)
Actinomycin D	16	2 (12.5%)	14 (87.5%)
Other chemotherapy (Single or multiple drugs)	47	16 (34.0%)	31 (66.0%)
No chemotherapy	168	70 (41.7%)	9 (58.3%)
Prior radiation therapy	140	52 (37.1%)	88 (62.9%)
No prior radiation therapy	127	49 (38.5%)	78 (61.5%)

thrombocytopenia in 167 patients (18.5%), overt bleeding in 87 (9.6%), death related to such bleeding in 50 (5.5%), and leukopenia in 58 (6.4%). Bleeding was often, although not always, associated with thrombocytopenia. Other abnormalities related to bleeding, such as poor clot retraction and prolonged prothrombin time and/or partial thromboplastin time, occurred but were not reported in sufficient number to provide valid data on their frequency. Fever, apparently due to the drug, was a common finding and was reported in 104 patients (11.5%). Decreased serum calcium was detected in 74 patients, but was not measured in many cases. Liver function tests were also abnormal in many patients in whom they were obtained, with 165 patients (18%) having an elevated SGOT. The Pfizer package insert recommends 25−30 mg/kg/day for 8−10 days given as a slow IV infusion over 6 h, stating that this dose produces less toxicity than 'push' injection. It urges that higher daily doses not be given.

Mackenzie et al. [54] administered mithramycin at 25−50 mg/kg/day for 3−10 days IV to 8 patients with disseminated testicular malignancies. Three patients obtained partial regressions, but two of the eight had hemorrhage without thrombocytopenia. None of the partial regressions were considered 'worthwhile' and the authors concluded. "Mithramycin should not be used except in patients with terminal disease, since its toxicity is unpredictable and other agents are more effective."

Ream et al. [76] also published a detailed study of mithramycin therapy. They administered the drug by constant IV infusion to 26 evaluable patients with testicular cancer, giving 25 mg/kg for 9−10 days in most cases. Nine of the 26 had objective responses, all in embryonal cell carcinomas with pulmonary metastases. Two of these patients had complete regressions. No response was seen in six patients with teratocarcinoma. One complete regression was of > 32 months duration while the other was > 12 months at the time of the report. Five of the seven patients having partial regressions were still alive but the duration of response was not given. Six patients with embryonal cell carcinoma had received actinomycin D plus methotrexate and/or chlorambucil prior to the mithramycin therapy, and five of them had shown no response to this therapy. After mithramycin therapy, one obtained a complete regression and two had > 50% response of extensive pulmonary metastases. Three patients failed to respond.

The toxic effects observed by Ream included nausea and vomiting in four patients, severe enough to require cessation of treatment in spite of the continuous infusion method, which the authors felt has much less gastrointestinal (GI) toxicity than rapid IV injection. Of the 26 patients, 25 had an increase in temperature during infusion, usually to about 38° C. Eight patients had bleeding episodes associated with drug administration, five of them without thrombocytopenia, but none died. Seven patients had erythema or an acneiform eruption near the end or several days after completion of a course. 'Modest' lever enzyme elevations occured regularly during the period of drug infusion but were reversible in all cases. Nine of the 20 patients evaluated developed a prothrombin time after treatment that was < 30% of the pretreatment level; three patients had abnormal clot retraction that was associated in two cases with bleeding in the absence of thrombocytopenia. Ream felt that a drop in the platelet count to greater than the pretreatment level, even if the count was still > 150,000, indicated a need for disontinuing therapy. He further stated "Vitamin K may correct the prolonged prothrombin time". He also recommended that because they may immediately precede development of a hemorrhagic diathesis epistaxis and dermatologic reactions are indications to stop mithramycin administration. In this series of patients, the optimum interval between courses was between 3 and 4 weeks.

Yarbo and Kennedy [120] have reported that mithramycin-treated liver cells in vitro rapidly recover their capacity in RNA synthesis but recovery is delayed in tumor cells. This finding suggested that an alternate-day dose regimen might reduce toxicity without altering antitumor activity. The clinical results of this schedule have been published by Kennedy [44] for 28 patients with testicular tumors treated with 50 mg/kg/dose. There was reportedly a reduction in the severity of toxicity, and "elimination of hemorrhage and mortality", while antitumor effect was retained with seven patients showing objective response.

Actinomycin D has not been investigated as extensively as mithramycin (Table 23). Mackenzie et al. [54] employed this antibiotic in 22 patients, obtaining five complete and five partial regressions. Dosage regimens used and responses seen are itemized in the following section for the 12 patients who received the drug as initial chemotherapy: (a) 1 mg/day × 5, by IV push [seven patients − two complete response (CR), two partial response (PR)]; (b) 1 mg/day × 4−5, by continuous IV infusion (two patients − one PR); (c) 0.25 mg/day × 22−32, by IV push (two patients − one CR, one failure later responding to treatment by continuous infusion); (d) 5 mg/day × 1, q 2 weeks, by IV push (one patient − no response). Ten patients received actinomycin D after prior treatment with other drugs, but only one responded.

Of the five patients who obtained complete regressions, four were alive and well at 11+, 19+, 20+, and 21+ months, and one was alive with recurrence at 9+ months. Two had embryonal cell carcinoma and three had teratocarcinoma. As the chemotherapy of choice for metastatic testicular tumors other than seminoma, Mackenzie et al. recommended 1 mg actinomycin D daily for 4−5 days, by IV push, at monthly intervals.

Tan et al. [101] treated one child having metastatic embryonal carcinoma with actinomycin D at a dose of 15 mg/kg/day for 5 days (IV) and obtained an objective response. Another child with the same diagnosis who received actinomycin D plus X-ray therapy did not respond.

Other antibiotics have also been reported to have activity against testicular tumors. Adriamycin, has significant activity (Table 24). Monfardini et al. [60] have reported activity in the range of 65% among 20 patients, including 15 carcinomas, mostly of the

Table 23. Actinomycin D therapy of testicular tumors

Reference no.	Dose schedule	No evaluable patients	No responses[a]		Response rate	
			CR	PR	CR	CR+PR
53	Various (a) 1.0 mg/day IV push × 5 days (b) 1.0 mg/day × 4–5 days by continuous infusion (c) 0.25 mg/day IV push × 22–32 days (d) 5 mg IV push every 2 weeks	22	5	5	23%	46%
101	15 µg/kg/day IV push × 5 days	2	–	1	–	50%

[a] CR, complete response; PR, partial response

Table 24. Adriamycin activity in testicular cancer

Reference no.	No. of evaluable points	No. of responses	Response rate (%)
60	20	13	65
68	12	2	17
9	5	1	20
100	2	1	50
	39	17	44

embryonal type. There were three responses among seminoma patients and one of these was a complete remission of 1-year's duration. In the carcinoma group, regressions occurred , in 10 of the 15 cases but there were no complete remissions.

Blum et al. [10] reported 57 evaluable patients with testicular carcinoma treated with bleomycin; 37 patients received the drug as a single agent and 20 were treated with bleomycin and vinblastine. The overall response was 32% for bleomycin alone and 90% for the combination. Responses were noted in all cell types but the duration of response again was short for both the single agent (1.5–2 months) and the combination (2–5 months).

Cis-diamminedichloroplatinum II (cisplatin) is the newest and probably the most active drug in testicular cancer. As a single agent, the drug has an overall response rate of 60% in 70 patients including 15 complete responders and 31 partial responders (Table 25). This is particularly impressive in a pretreated population. The most common single agent regimen used was 20 mg/m²/day for 5 days repeated at 4-week intervals. Moderate myelosuppression and transient increases in serum creatinine were repeated.

Table 25. Cisplatin in the treatment of testicular cancer

Reference	No. of evaluable points	No. of responses		Response rate	
		CR	PR	CR	CR+PR
37	9	0	6	0	66
59	10	6	3	60	90
38	15	7	3	47	66
67	2	0	1	0	50
70	22	1	14	4	68
77	12	1	4	8	42
Total	70	15	31	21	66

In summary, testicular tumors appear to be responsive to a wide range of single agents. Drugs such as cisplatin, vinblastine, bleomycin, mithramycin, actinomycin D, and phenylalanine mustard appear to induce a significant number of remissions. No chemotherapeutic agent adequately evaluated has been established as completely inactive.

Combination Chemotherapy

It is interesting to note that the concept of combining antitumor drugs, which has proven so valuable in the hematologic malignancies, had one of its first applications more than a decade ago in testicular tumors.

a. "Triple Therapy":

In 1960, Li et al. [50] published the first account of treatment with a three-drug combination in metastatic testicular cancer (Table 26). This report and a subsequent one [49] employed a regimen of chlorambucil (10 mg/day PO for 16−25 days), actinomycin D (0.5 mg/day IV on days 3−7, 12−16, and 21−25), and methotrexate 5 mg/day PO for 16−25 days. Maintenance therapy varied, but in general was summarized as follows: "Once every 2 weeks for two courses, once monthly until all objective evidences of disease have disappeared and once every two months thereafter . . . Each course of therapy consists of chlorambucil and methotrexate in combination for seven days plus a five day course of actinomycin D beginning on the third day". Among 28 patients treated, there were ten complete and four partial remissions; at least one of the complete responses occurred in a patient with choriocarcinoma. Li felt that the efficacy of the triple-drug regimen was superior to his results with chlorambucil alone of chlorambucil plus methotrexate (response in one of nine patients), 6-mercaptopurine plus L-6-diazo-5-oxo-norleucine (response in one of eight patients), or an alkylating agent plus actinomycin D (response in two of nine patients). Of the 14 responders on triple-drug therapy, two were alive and free of disease at the time of Li's second report [49], seven alive but in relapse, and five had died following relapse. No data were given on the median duration of remission, but the first report cited a range of 1−18+ months.

There is scanty discussion of toxicity in Li's two reports. In the first he stated that "drug toxicity as manifested by nausea, vomiting, weakness, stomatitis, diarrhea, leuko-

Table 26. Triple drug therapy in testicular tumors[a]

Reference	No. evaluable patients	No. responses[b]		Response rate	
		CR	PR	CR	CR+PR
49, 50	28	10	4	36%	50%
111	90	11	26	12%	41%
53	29	–	11	–	39%
5	11	1	4	9%	45%
CTEP[c]	44	1	15	2%	34%
	202	23	60	11%	41%

[a] Regimen: Actinomycin D − 0.5 mg/day IV day 3−7, day 12−16, day 21−25; Chlorambucil − 10 mg/day PO × 16−25; Methotrexate − 5 mg/day PO × 16−25

[b] CR, complete response; PR, partial response

[c] Unpublished data on file in Cancer Therapy Evaluation Program, Division of Cancer Treatment, NCI

All drugs given as 5-day courses

penia, thrombocytopenia, acneiform skin eruptions, and moderate loss of hair was extremely variable from patient to patient. . . Actinomycin D could possibly augment a pre-existing radiation reaction and could contribute to increasing pulmonary insufficiency; such as was the case in (one) patient. . . who rapidly died of respiratory failure with little evidence of metastatic disease in the lungs but with diffuse pulmonary fibrosis". No other deaths associated with drug toxicity were mentioned.

In his second report, Li stated that "recovery from drug toxicity generally takes 7−14 days", and advised temperary discontinuation of triple therapy when stomatitis, diarrhea, a WBC < 3,000, or platelet count < 100,000 are first noted. Treatment was not to be reinstituted "until full recovery. . . is obtained". No specific breakdown was offered as to the type and extent of toxicity.

In another application of triple therapy, Whitmore (111) reported objective responses in three patients with seminomas, in 17 of 25 with embryonal cell carcinoma, in 11 of 17 teratocarcinomas, and in seven of ten choriocarcinomas. He stated that "the regression was of no practical value in most instances, either because of its brevity or because of its in completeness". However, he noted long-term disease-free survivals of 9+, 33+, and 42+ months in three patients. Each of these patients had pulmonary metastases before treatment, and one (the 42+ months survivor) had choriocarcinoma. The other two had embryonal cell carcinoma. If would seem that the practical value of the regression in these three patients was great indeed. Interestingly, Whitmore also cited survivals of 36+ and 75+ months, respectively, in one patient with choriocarcinoma who received actinomycin D and chlorambucil and another with teratocarcinoma who received 6-MP and DON. The latter, however, had only an elevated urinary HCG level as evidence of disease prior to treatment.

Mackenzie [53] has also reported the use of triple-drug therapy, essentially as administered by Li, in 90 cases of metastatic testicular cancer that yielded 11 CR and 26 PR. The group included 72 patients who received the three agents as their primary chemotherapy; ten of the CR occurred in these patients and the overall response rate was 50%. Five of the complete responders were alive and well at the time of the report, at intervals of 24+, 53+, 55+, 77+, and 85+ months; two of them had a primary diagnosis of choriocarcinoma, two had embryonal cell tumors, and one had teratocarcinoma. The six deaths in the complete response group occurred at 7, 17, 18, 19, 25, and 29 months (median = 18.5 months); five had embryonal cell carcinoma and one had choriocarcinoma. Mackenzie did not specifically discuss the toxicity encountered in this series.

Astrakhan and Monul [5] have described the results of combined chemotherapy in testicular tumors resistant to phenylalanine mustard and X irradiation. Actinomycin D, methotrexate, and (apparently) chloramabucil were used but the doses were unclear. Of 29 patients, 11 experienced objective improvement but no responses were obtained in chorionepitheliomas (presumably choriocarcinomas) or in teratoblastomas. Side effects included leukopenia, thrombocytopenia, and 'dyseptic disorders', without further details.

Moore [61] has published a study of 11 patients treated by Li's method, except that 5-day maintenance courses were given every month using each drug in the same dose employed in the initial therapy. Ten of the patients had embryonal cell carcinoma and/or teratocarcinoma, and one had choriocarcinoma. One patient obtained complete remission and was alive and apparently disease-free at 54+ months. Four patients showed prolonged improvement, while three had only transient improvement and three failed to respond at all. Mean survivals were 6 months for the nonresponders, 9 months for temporary responders, and 22 months for prolonged responders, excluding the single apparent 'cure'.

A variety of other two- and three-drug approaches are outlined in Table 27. Mackenzie et al. [54] used actinomycin D plus chlorambucil in 31 patients with testicular tumors, giving the drugs as in 'triple therapy' but with the deletion of methotrexate. Five patients had CR and eight had partial regressions. Two of the complete responders were alive and well at 17+ and 47+ months; two were alive with recurrence at 35+ and 37+ months and one was dead after 64 months. Two of the complete responders had choriocarcinoma, two had embryonal cell carcinoma, and one had teratocarcinoma. All 13 of the responses were in patients who had not received previous chemotherapy. No details were given concerning toxicity.

Jacobs et al. [41] reported on the use of three forms of combination therapy: (1) mechlorethamine alternating on a monthly basis with actinomycin D; (2) mechlorethamine alternating on a monthly basis with methotrexate; and (3) vincristine plus methotrexate plus phenylalanine mustard or cyclophosphamide, with the latter two drugs given as 'tolerated'. Mechlorethamine plus actinomycin D produced three reponses in six cases of embryonal cell carcinoma, no response in one case of teratocarcinoma, and one reponse among seven patients with mixed cell tumors; durations were 1, 1, and 78+ months for the embryonal cell patients and 4 months for the mixed cell responder. Mechlorethamine plus methotrexate gave responses in three of seven cases of embryonal cell carcinomas, one of four teratocarcinomas, and one in four mixed tumors, with durations of 21, 3, 18, 28+, and 40+ months (the longest was in the teratocarcinoma patient). Therapy with the three-drug combination produced responses in one of two embryonal cell carcinomas, in three of eight mixed tumors, and no responses in two teratocarcinomas; durations were 3, 4, 5, and 5 months, respectively. Toxicity was minimal in all three regimens. The lowest white cell count was 2,000 and there was no life-threatening episode of any kind.

Steinfeld et al. [97] tested a combination of vincristine, methotrexate, and phenylalanine mustard in 12 evaluable patients with advanced metastatic germinal tumors. Vincristine was administered at 0.05 mg/kg/week (= 1.85 mg/m^2/week),

Table 27. Other two- and three-drug combination therapy in testicular tumors

Reference	Dose schedule	No. evaluable patients	No. responses[a]		Response rate	
			Cr	PR	CR	CR+PR
54	Actinomycin D 0.5 mg/day IV, days 3–7, 12–16, 21–25 + Chlorambucil 10 mg/day PO × 16–25	31	5	8	16%	42%
41	Mechlorethamine 0.4 mg/kg × 1 IV, months 1, 3, 5, 7, etc. + Actinomycin D 0.5 mg/day × 4 IV, months 2, 4, 6, etc.	14	1	3	7%	29%
	Mechlorethamine 0.4 mg/kg × 1 IV, months 1, 3, 5, 7, etc. + Methotrexate 25 mg/day × 5 IV, months 2, 4, 6, 8 etc.	15	2	3	13%	33%
97	1. Vincristine 0.05 mg/kg week 2. Methotrexate 5 mg/day PO 3. Phenylalanine mustard 0.075 mg/kg/day PO	12	1	8	8%	75%
41	As in [41] except cyclophosphamide (2 mg/kg/day PO) substituted for phenylalanine mustard	12	–	4	–	334

[a] *CR*, complete response; *PR*, partial response

methotrexate at 5 mg/day PO, and phenylalanine mustard at 0.075 mg/kg/day (2.8 mg/m^2/day); all three drugs were administered to 'limiting toxicity'. Objective regressions were noted in three of four evaluable seminomas, one of which was a CR lasting 959+ days, and in each of two choriocarcinomas lasting 314+ days and 1,218+ days. One of the latter had successful resection of cerebral metastases after an unsuccessful course of intrathecal methotrexate. Regressions lasting 33–160 days (median 50 days) also occurred in four of six embryonal cell carcinomas. Overall, 9 of 12 patients experienced marked responses although they were short-lived.
The 'most objectionable' toxicity was due to vincristine, with severe peripheral neuropathy, abdominal pain, and constipation supervening in many patients. Thrombocytopenia often forced a decrease in the dose of phenylalanine mustard and/or methotrexate; five patients had platelet counts below 50,000. Six patients had white cell counts (WBC) > 1,500 on therapy, five of them developing this leukopenia

Table 28. Four-drug combination therapy in testicular tumors

Reference	Dose schedule	No. evaluable patients	No. responses		Response rate	
			CR	PR	CR	CR+PR
40	1. Vincristine 0.025 mg/ kg/week 2. Actinomycin D 2 mg every other week alternated with 3. Mithramycin 50 by 6 h infusion every other week 4. Cyclophosphamide 2 mg/ kg/day PO	7	3	2	42%	71%
58	1. 5-Fluorouracil 7.5 mg/kg/ day × 5 2. Cyclophosphamide 7.5 mg/ kg/day, days 1 and 4 3. Methotraxate 0.75 mg/ kg/day, days 1 and 4 4. Vincristine 0.025 mg/ kg/day, days 1 and 4	17	5	2	29%	41%

within 35 days of the start of treatment. The hematocrit dropped 6% or more in 13 patients, often before 2 weeks of treatment had been completed.

Because of the severity of the vincristine toxicity in Steinfeld's series and the known platelet sparing effect of cyclophosphamide, Solomon et al. [92] tried a somewhat different three-drug combination. The vincristine dose was reduced to 0.025 mg/kg. These drugs were continued as long as possible and doses were adjusted as tolerated. In embryonal cell carcinoma, five of eight patients had a PR with a median duration of 63 days. There was no response in one patient with choriocarcinoma but one seminoma exhibited a PR lasting 84 days. Of 25 patients evaluable for toxic effects, including tumor types other than testicular, 60% developed at WBC < 1,500, 28% had platelets < 50,000, and 16% had hemorrhage associated with thrombocytopenia. Anemia developed in 24% and was severe enough to require transfusion; 52% experienced nausea, vomiting, anorexia, and stomatitis; 80% developed some evidence of peripheral neuropathy, and 32% were constipated. The authors concluded that this type of combination therapy was effective, but "early relapses . . . were disappointing and appeared to be related to the high incidence of adverse drug reactions which necessitated reductions in dose".

Two older attempts at therapy with four-drug combinations have been reported (Table 28). Jacobs [40] alternated mithramycin with actinomycin D combined with cyclophosphamide and vincristine, but the numbers were too small to draw a definitive conclusion. Mendelson [58] treated 17 patients with a four-drug combination of 5-fluorouracil (5-FU), cyclophosphamide, methotrexate, and vincristine. He reported that "subsequent courses were given after the nadir of leukopenia and when marrow recovery was evident (usually (10−14 days). The mean number of courses required to achieve a CR was 2.8. Remissions were maintained with a course of drugs once every

Table 29. Vinblastine and bleomycin protocols in testicular cancer at M.D. Anderson Hospital [80−82]

VB−I	Velban 0.4 mg/kg total dose, days 1 and 2 Bleomycin 30 units IM twice weekly × 10 weeks Additional courses of Velban unchanged Bleomycin 30 units IM twice weekly × 5 weeks; Repeat at 4-week intervals
VB−2	Bleomycin 30 units/liter normal saline over 24 h × 5 days Velban 0.4 mg/kg days 5 and 6
VB−3	Velban 0.4−0.6 mg/kg days 1 and 2 Bleomycin 30 units/liter normal saline over 24 h × 5 days (days 2 through 6)
VB−3 + sequential cis-platinum	Add cis-platinum 100 mg/m^2 upon recovery from myelosuppression × 2 at 7-day intervals

two months". Five of the 17 patients had CRs with a range of 5−52+ months and a mean duration of 13.8 months. Two others experienced partial remissions of 3 months and 2 weeks, respectively. Accompanying toxicity was reported as 'mild'; leukopenia occurred regularly but a WBC below 2,000 was not observed.

Modern Era Combination Chemotherapy

The modern era of combination chemotherapy in testicular cancer begins with the core combination of vinblastine and bleomycin. This combination was first studied at M.D. Anderson Hospital and their experience ranges over three protocols (Table 29). The response rate on these protocols plus two studies of the Southwest Oncology Group are outlined on Table 30.

Samuels et al. [81] first combined bleomycin with vinblastine for the therapy of testicular tumors, as follows: Bleomycin 15 mg IM was administered twice weekly for 5 weeks and vinblastine was given at 0.4−0.6 mg/kg IV in two fractions (days 1 and 2). Fifty patients were treated according to this induction scheme, and if a response was seen additional therapy consisting of three or four courses of the same vinblastine dose and 50% of the dose of bleomycin was given. Sixteen patients achieved complete remission (CR; 32%) with this regimen, and 15 were free of disease after 2 years. Twenty-two other patients experienced partial remission (PR; > 50% reduction in maximum tumor diameter), with a median survival of 32 weeks. Five patients developed interstitial pneumonitis secondary to bleomycin therapy.

Samuels et al. [80] then modified their approach to a regimen in which vinblastine was given at 0.4 mg/kg in two fractions (days 1 and 2) and bleomycin (30 mg in 1,000 ml 5% D/W over 24 h) was started on day 2 for five additional days. Courses were repeated every 21−28 days for three or four courses. Forty stage III germinal tumors and four extragonadonal primary tumors were studied. In 39 evaluable patients with high tumor volume presentations there were 19 with CR (47%) and ten with PR. In the extragonadal group, one CR and one PR were seen. The mean survival of complete responders was 34 weeks with none dead. Toxicity included severe leukopenia in 40

Table 30. Vinblastine plus bleomycin at MD Anderson for treatment of testicular cancer

Regimen [Reference]	Doses mg/m^2		No. of evaluable points	% CR	% CR+PR
	Vinblastine	Bleomycin			
VB−1 [80, 81]	0.2−0.3 mg/kg day 1 and 2	30 units twice weekly IM	51	33	70
VB−2 [80, 81]	0.2−0.3 mg/kg day 5 and 6	30 units/day × 5, continuous IV infusion	3	33	100
VB−3 [82]	0.2−0.3 mg/kg day 1 and 2	30 units/day × 5, continuous IV infusion	91	65	94
SWOG VB−1 modification [94]	0.2 mg/kg day 1 and 2	15 units/m^2 twice weekly IV	11	45	82
SWOG Controlled study modification of VB−1 [93]	16 mg/m^2 day 1 and 2 IV	15 units/m^2 twice weekly	48	44	65

patients, thrombocytopenia in 21, hemolytic anemia in 13, stomatitis in all cases, and bleomycin pneumonitis in two.

Samuels [81] compared his experience with Velban plus biweekly bleomycin in 26 patients with that recorded in 34 patients who received Velban plus continuous bleomycin. In the biweekly bleomycin group, seven (20%) achieved CR, as against 21 (61%) with the continuous infusion approach. The median survival was also superior in the latter group (78+ weeks as against 48 weeks). These data, Samuels feels, show the clear-cut advantage for the infusion approach with bleomycin.

In a more recent paper, Samuels et al. have reported on 99 patients who were entered on the VB-3 protocol between July 1, 1973, and January 31, 1977 [82]. Only 5% of these patients wee classified as III-A or III-B-I in a clinical classification of stage III patients (Table 31). Of the patients, 75% had advanced disease (III-B-3, B-4, B-5). The histology was evenly distribution between embryonal carcinoma (45%) and teratocarcinoma (45%) with 10% being choriocarcinoma. Forty-three of the patients were failed stage III patients who had undergone prior retroperitoneal node dissection and radiotherapy.

Ninety-one patients were deemed evaluable and CR was recorded in 59 (65%). This was equivalent for all histologic types. Patients with minimal disease and embryonal carcinoma had a 100% CR rate with 92% having no evidence of disease (NED). In this good risk group, prior radiotherapy did not exert a deleterious effect. In patients with advanced disease, previously irradiated patients had only a 50% CR rate. Three of these ultimately failed so that the salvage rate for advanced disease patients with prior X-ray treatment was only 20%. For patients with advanced disease and no prior radiotherapy, the CR rate was 56% with only one failure.

Table 31. Stratification of stage III testicular carcinoma patients at M.D. Anderson Hospital

III–A	Disease confined to supraclavicular nodes
III–B–1	Gynecomastia, either unilateral or bilateral with or without elevation of biomarkers. Estrogen levels may be elevated. No gross tumor detectable.
III–B–2	Minimal pulmonary disease. Up to five metastatic masses in each lung, with largest diameter of any single lesion no greater than 2.0 cm
III–B–3	Advanced pulmonary disease. Any mediastinal or hilar mass, neoplastic pleural effusion, or intrapulmonary mass greater than 2.0 cm in diameter
III–B–4	Advanced abdominal disease. Any palpable abdominal mass, ureteral displacement or obstructive uropathy
III–B–5	Visceral disease (excluding lung), most commonly the liver, also gastrointestinal tract and brain

Table 32. Response and survival rates according to Velban dose in VB–3 study at M.D. Anderson Hospital

Velban dose (mg/kg)	No. of patients	No. receiving prior X-ray therapy	No. CR	% CR	No. CR surviving
< 0.4	24	18	9	38	6
0.4–0.45	49	18	28	57	20
0.5	14	6	12	86	12
≥ 0.6	12	1	10	83	9
93	43	59	60	47	

In teratocarcinoma patients, the CR rate in minimal disease patients was 80% with three subsequent failures for a salvage rate of only 50%. The numbers are too small to reflect a radiotherapy effect.

The Velban dosage correlated with CR and salvage (Table 32). At the lowest Velban dose (< 0.4 mg/kg), there was only a 38% CR rate, with 33% of these relapsing. At the next level (0.4–0.45 mg/kg), this increased to 57% with 29% of these failing. As the Velban dose went up to 0.5 mg/kg or greater, the CR rate jumbed to 85% with only one failure.

Cis-platinum was used as primary induction therapy in nine patients and as secondary therapy for VB-3 failures in 16. In the primary group, eight achieved CR and are all disease-free. Eight of these patients had advanced presentation. Of the 16 VB-3 failures treated with cis-platinum, nine had achieved a prior CR and complete stable responses were reinduced in two, with four achieving only a PR. These latter four patients then underwent thoractomy and all were in stable remission after 18 months.

The major dose-limiting toxicity was leukopenia. With low-dose Velban, septicemia was observed in 2.3% of the drug courses. With higher doses of Velban (≥ 0.5 mg/kg) this increased to 9.2% with one death. This increase is primarily due to the increased severity of the stomatitis, acneiform skin reactions, and paralytic ileus. In this situation, meticulous attention to oral hygiene, skin care, fluid balance, and antibiotic administration is obligatory.

The mean dose of bleomycin was 10 above 700 mg. Bleomycin-induced interstitial pneumonitis was seen in only two cases and both recovered. Three patients presented with hypersensitivity pneumonitis induced by bleomycin and all responded to corticosteriod therapy.

The Velban-bleomycin combination has been used as adjuvant therapy in 27 patients with stage II disease after lymphadnectomy. Twenty-one of these had gross disease in which the surgeon could identify tumor at the time of operation. Six had only microscopically demonstrated disease. Six were treated with the VB-1 regimen, 19 with VB-3 and 2 with bleomycin-COMF. The original intention was to treat with four adjuvant courses. In four cases, more than four courses were given and one patient each received two and three courses only. The courses were given at full doses with the Velban dose being 0.4–0.6 mg/kg. The highest doses were given to those with residual tumor after surgery and with choriocarcinoma. The lowest doses were given to patients with prior irradiation.

In the 21 cases with gross disease, 18 continue to have NED with a mean survival of 125 weeks. Three patients have died. Of the six with microscopic disease, all have NED with a mean survival of 225 weeks. Therefore, 24/27 still remain disease-free with a mean survival of 144 weeks. The major toxicity with this adjuvant regimen is leukopenia. Virtually all patients developed a severe but short-lived depression in leukocytes to less than 1,000 mm^3. The nadir was usually seen between days 6 and 8 with recovery by days 12–14. Stomatitis was observed in all patients treated. Two patients developed sepsis and one died. One case of bleomycin pulmonary toxicity was seen with recovery.

Five patients with stage III disease after thoractomy (four cases) and laparatomy (one case) were also treated with these adjuvant regimens and four remain disease-free.

At the Memorial Sloan-Kettering Cancer Center, a series of regimens evolved from the nucleus of vinblastine and bleomycin (Table 33) [35].

The first regimen (VAB I) involved daily doses of a three-drug combination of bleomycin (0.4 mg/kg), actinomycin D (0.0075–0.015 mg/kg), and vinblastine (0.025–0.05 mg/kg) [86]. Each drug was given IV on days 1, 2, and 3, and repeated for two or three doses in 7–14 days as toxicity permitted. Twenty-one patients were treated and 16 were evaluabale; of these, eight showed objective responses lasting 1–5 months. Hematologic toxicity was predictable and mucocutaneous toxicity between days 4 and 20 was frequently severe and dose-limiting. Pulmonary toxicity was observed in one patient.

The VAB II regimen [18] consisted of the following: Bleomycin by IV infusion of 0.5 mg/kg/day for 7 days, vinblastine 0.06 mg/kg and actinomycin D 0.02 mg/kg on day 1, and platinum 1 mg/kg on day 8. Maintenance was with vinblastine, actinomycin, and bleomycin once weekly, with platinum substituting for actinomycin every 3rd week. The induction course was repeated 4 months after the start of therapy. Following this reinduction, maintenance was changed to vinblastine 0.1 mg/kg and actinomycin 0.025 mg/kg every 3 weeks and chlorambucil 0.1 mg/kg PO daily for a total of 2–3 years in the absence of relapse.

Of 50 patients treated with VAB II regimen, 25 (50%) achieved CR and 17 (34%) PR. Tumor shrinkage began within 2 weeks. The median duration of response was 13

Table 33. The VAB regimens of Memorial Hospital for testicular cancer [35]

Regimen	Vinblastine	Bleomycin	Actinomycin D	Other drugs	No. evaluable points	% CR	% of those originally entered with NED
VAB	0.025−0.05 All drugs given days 1, 2, 3, 9, 10, 11, then weekly maintenance: VLB 0.05−0.10 mg/kg; ACTD 0.015−0.03 mg/kg; Bleo 0.1−0.25 units/kg	0.40 units/kg	0.0075−0.015 mg/kg		71	14	12
VAB II	0.06 mg/kg day 1 Repeat every 3 months Maintenance: VLB, ACTD, BLEO weekly; Platinum replaces ACTD every 3 weeks	0.5 units/kg/day day 1−7 continuous IV	0.02 mg/kg day 1	Platinum 1 mg/kg day 8	50	50	22
VAB III	0.4 mg/m^2 days 1 Repeat every 4−5 months Maintenance (21-day cycle): VLB 4 mg/m^2 every 3 weeks; chlorambucil 4 mg/m^2 day 1−14 PO; ACTD 1 mg/m^2; Adriamycin 45 mg/m^2 alternate; Platinum 50 mg/m^2 every 3 weeks	200/m^2 day 1−7 continuous infusion IV	1 mg/m^2 day 1	Platinum 120 mg/m^2 day 8; Cytoxan 600 mg/m^2 day 1	90	60	49

VLB, vinblatine; *ACTD*, actinomycin D; *Bleo*, bleomycin

months for the CR group but only 5 months for the PR group. In the CR group, 23 patients became free of measurable disease on chemotherapy alone; two additional patients had surgery at a later date because of residual disease after chemotherapy. At the time of the recent literature report, the mediansurvival for the CR group has not yet been reached, with 11 patients still disease-free at 16–33 months. All those not achieving CR had a median survival of only 9 months. In patients without previous chemotherapy, the CR rate was 60%, with a median duration of 21 months. In those with prior drug treatment, the CR rate was 40% with only an 8-month median duration.

Nausea and vomiting caused by actinomycin and platinum were universal and lasted for at least 1–2 days, occasionally for a long as 1–2 weeks, especially after platimum. Mucositis and alopecia occurred in most patients. Fewer than 15% of the patients had a leukopenia value below 3,000, and all of these had had prior radiation and/or chemotherapy. Platelet counts of less than 100,000 were seen in only one patient. There were no cases of drug-related sepsis. Of the patients, 20% had transient elevation of serum creatinine to greater than 2.0 mg/100 ml. There was one bleomycin-related death from progressive pulmonary insufficiency, occurring 5 days after an abdominal operation during which high oxygen concentration was used. A modest decrease in vital capacity by 10%–20% of the baseline value was common.

VAB III [2] consists of bleomycin given by continuous infusion (20 mg/m^2), cyclophosphamide (600 mg/m^2), and actinomycin D (1 mg/m^2). High-dose cis-platinum diammine dichloride (120 mg/m^2) is given on day 8, with prehydration and a sustained mannitol diuresis. Maintenance with Velban (4 mg/m^2) every 3 weeks and chlorambucil 4 mg/m^2 PO daily is given for 2 of every 3 weeks. Actinomycin D (1 mg/m^2), adriamycin (45 mg/m^2), and platinum (50 mg/m^2) are alternated. The induction phase is repeated at 4- to 5-month intervals. In 90 evaluable patients, the CR rate was reported as 60%, with 49% showing NED [35].

In the VAB IV regimen, a second course of treatment without bleomycin is given 16 weeks after the start of chemotherapy, and a third course with all the drugs is given at 32 weeks. This regimen has produced CR in 29 of 55 patients, and 11 more were made free of disease by operation. Seven have relapsed so that in the last report 60% remained disease-free.

The most recent (VAB-6) protocol [106] has evolved from lessons learned from the earlier VAB studies. These lessons have been summarized as follows: (1) Induction is the most effective part of treatment; (2) long maintenance is probably not required; (3) bulky metastases frequently have incomplete regression; (4) long-term complete remission can be achieved with complete resection of residual tumor and additional chemotherapy.

The VAB-6 protocol is outlined in Table 34. To date, CRs have been observed in 19/21 (90%) treated with this induction regimen. These patients had either stage III or unresectable stage II disease and no prior chemotherapy exposure. One relapse has occurred to date.

Einhorn [27 and Einhorn and Donahue [29] have reported on 50 patients with germ-cell tumors of the testes, with metastatic measurable disease, treated with a regimen called PVB. Platinum 20 mg/m^2/day for 5 days was given as a 15-min IV infusion. The platinum was repeated every 3 weeks for three courses. Vinblastine was given on days 1 and 2 in a total dosage of 0.4 mg/kg for a total of five courses and then given as a single injection in a dosage of 0.3 mg/kg every 4 weeks for a total of 2 years

Table 34. The VAB-6 protocol of Memorial Hospital

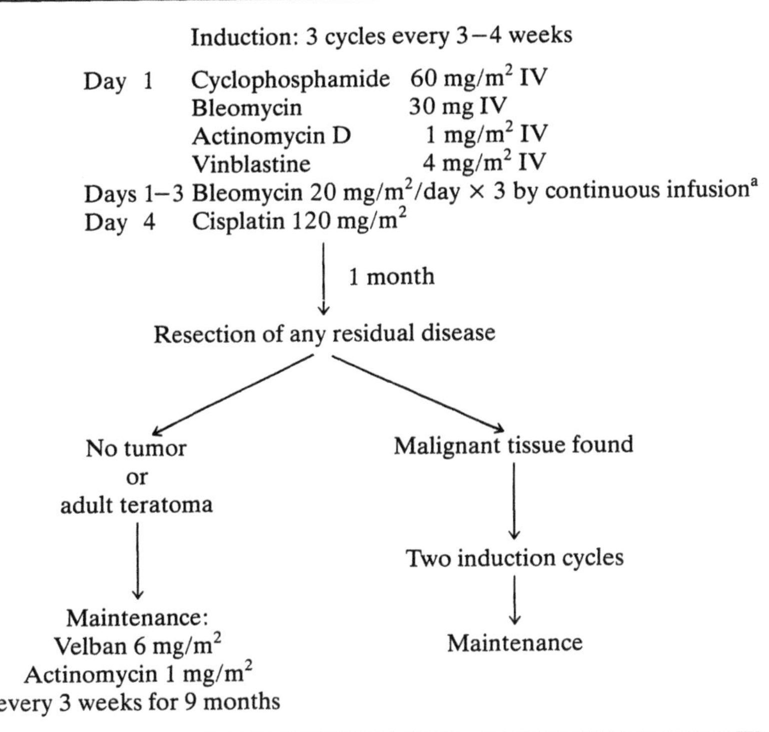

ᵃ Omitted on 3rd cycle

of therapy. Bleomycin, 30 units IV, was given on days 2, 9, and 16 of each platinum course, and was given with the platinum 6 h after the vinblastine and then weekly for a total of 13 weeks. The bleomycin was stopped at a total dosage of 350 units to minimize pulmonary fibrosis. "Fifty patients were studied initially. Thirty-three of 47 evaluable patients (71%) achieved complete remission. Only five of these 33 complete remissions have relapsed at the last report. In addition, five of the twelve partial remissions were rendered disease-free following surgical removal of residual disease after significant reduction of tumor volume with chemotherapy".

The platinum caused moderate to severe nausea and vomiting in all patients during each 5-day course. Vigorous hydration has been used, 100 cm³ normal saline/h being given for 12 h before administration of the drug and then a continuous drip at 100 cm³/h throughout the 5 days of the platinum dosing. With this approach, biochemical manifestations of renal toxicity have been uncommon in Einhorn's experience.

Bleomycin in the regimen has produced fever, chills, and skin toxicity, none of which caused dose modification. All patients had significant alopecia and most had weight loss. The average weight loss was 20 lb. There was one death in the 50 patients from pulmonary fibrosis.

The most serious side effect was leukopenia, which was seen in all patients. The nadir was usually 1,000 between days 7 and 14. Eighteen patients required hospitalization

Table 35. PVB $\pm$ Adriamycin at University of Indiana 1976–1978

Regimen	No. of patients	No. CR	% CR	% CR+PR	% NED with surgery	% continuously NED
PVB (0.4)	26	18	69	100	19	69
PVB (0.3)	27	17	63	100	15	67
PVB + Adriamycin	25	18	72	92	8	68
	78	53	68	98	14	68

for presumed sepsis with granulocytopenic fever. Seven had documented gram-negative sepsis and one of these patients died of sepsis.

Einhorn follows patients postoperatively once a month for the first year with chest X-rays and beta-HCG and alpha-fetoprotein determinations. He feels this allows him to pick up relapse with minimal disease being present. In such patients, he has achieved CR in 20/22.

A second study was then undertaken by Williams and Einhorn [115] to attempt to reduce toxicity without impairing therapeutic response. In this study, the original PVB regimen was compared to the same regimen with the vinblastine dose lowered to 0.3 mg/kg. A third arm added Adriamycin to the PVB combination. The results to date (Table 35) show no difference in complete remission rate or disease-free status between the three treatment arms. The patients receiving the low-dose vinblastine arm had the fewest episodes of granulocytopenic fever.

When the two studies of Einhorn et al. are put together, the data indicate that prior therapy (Table 36) and extent of disease (Table 37) are important prognostic variables.

Recently, at Stanford [46], an analysis was undertaken of the severe marrow toxicity that can result after vinblastine, bleomycin, and platinum. The analysis showed that severe marrow toxicity was strongly correlated with Karnofsky performance status and prior exposure to radiation. In view of this, a sliding scale of vinblastine dosage based on these two features has been developed (Table 38). This has been incorporated into a current Northern California Oncology Group protocol.

The Southwest Oncology Group [78] has studied the PVB regimen in 126 patients. The doses are as follows: Vinblastine 12 mg/m^2 D1, 29 etc.; bleomycin 15 units/m^2 twice weekly until a total dose of 200 units/m^2 is reached; cisplatin 15 mg/m^2 D1–5, 29–33 etc.

This induction period lasts four months. Patients in CR or then receive a maintenance regimen as follows: Actinomycin D 1.5 mg/m^2 D1, 58 etc.; chlorambucil 10 mg/m^2 PO D4–8, 61–66 etc.; vinblastine 12 mg/m^2 D29, 87 etc.

The maintenance lasts for a total of 20 months giving 2 years of total therapy. If there was prior irradiation to more than 25% of the bone-marrow-bearing areas, then the initial vinblastine dose was lowered to 9 mg/m^2.

In the 126 patients so treated, there were 64 CRs (51%) and 33 PRs (26%). The CR rate broken down by cell type shows the highest rate to be with embryonal carcinomas where it was 71% (37/52). In pure seminomas, it was 2/8, teratoma 2/4, and choriocarcinoma 1/4. In 26 teratocarcinomas, ten (38%) achieved more CR. In

Table 36. Prior therapy and response to PVB Adriamycin derived from Einhorn

	No. of patients	No. CR	%
Surgery alone	73	48	65
Prior chemotherapy	36	27	75
Prior radiotherapy	18	14	77
Prior radiotherapy + chemotherapy	4	1	25

Table 37. Extent of disease and response to PVB Adriamycin derived from Einhorn

	No. of patients	No. CR	% CR
Minimal pulmonary disease	24	21	87
Advanced pulmonary disease	29	16	55
Minimal abdominal and pulmonary disease	22	21	95
Advanced abdominal disease	39	18	46
Elevated markers only	7	7	100
Miscellaneous	4	3	75

Table 38. Vinblastine dosage

No prior therapeutic experience with radiation or other chemotherapy program		Prior exposure to radiation or other chemotherapy program	
Karnofsky	Vinblastine dose (days 1 and 2)	Karnofsky	Vinblastine dose (days 1 and 2)
K = 50%	0.13 mg/kg	K = 50%	0.11 mg/kg
K = 60%	0.14 mg/kg	K = 60%	0.12 mg/kg
K = 70%	0.15 mg/kg	K = 70%	0.13 mg/kg
K = 80%	0.16 mg/kg	K = 80%	0.14 mg/kg
K = 90%	0.17 mg/kg	K = 90%	0.15 mg/kg
K = 100%	0.18 mg/kg	K = 100%	0.16 mg/kg

20 patients who had choriocarcinoma mixed with other cell types seven were observed to have a CR (35%).

In the 64 CRs, seven (11%) have relapsed at the median of 5 months. The median duration of CR in all 64 patients is now in excess of 1 year. For partial responders it is 4 months. At the time of the literature report, only 12 (19%) of the complete responders were in remission for more than 1 year indicating the early nature of the study.

Marrow toxicity was dose-limiting. Leukopenia below 3,000 cells/mm^3 was noted in 57% of evaluable courses and thrombocytopenia below 100,000 cells/mm^3 in 18%. There was one toxic death. There was one case of bilateral pulmonary fibrosis with pulmonary insufficiency due to bleomycin.

Einhorn [28] has recently summarized his group's surgical experience after induction with the VBP regimen. Twenty patients underwent thoractomy for resection of residual pulmonary metastases. Of these, eight were found to have only benign mature teratoma and four had necrotic fibrous tissue. Ten of these 12 have remained disease-free with two of the patients with necrotic fibrous tissues subsequently developing brain metastases. The remaining eight patients had residual tumor resected and only one remains disease-free. A total of 40 patients underwent laparatomy for retroperitioneal node dissection. This was undertaken only when all pulmonary disease had cleared but residual abdominal disease remained. Twenty-seven patients had either benign mature teratoma [12] or fibrous tissues [15] remaining and all remain disease-free, including two with teratomas who relapsed but were induced again with drugs. In the 13 patients who had all visible malignant tissues removed, three remain disease-free, along with two who are disease-free following salvage drug treatment after relapse. It is clear that those who demonstrate malignant disease at surgery require continued aggressive therapy.

Sogani et al. [91] have reviewed the surgery experience at the Memorial Sloan-Kettering Cancer Center after two or three induction courses of the VAB (IV–VI) protocols. A total of 39 patients were treated with the sequential chemotherapy followed by surgery. In 27 patients, the residual disease found at surgery could be completely resected. These broke down into 11 patients with no residual tumor found, eight with adult teratoma, and eight with residual malignant disease. In the first group, 10 of 11 patients are still disease-free. In the eight patients with teratoma, only one has relapsed. Eight patients with residual malignant disease were given more chemotherapy after surgery and seven are alive and in CR. In 12 patients, complete resection was not possible and in spite of continued drug treatment, none was made tumor-free. Complete excision of the residual disease following combination chemotherapy appears to be the most important prognostic factor with 24 of 27 patients in that category still alive without disease.

A cautionary note about cytoreductive surgery has been sounded by Lange et al. [47]. They have reported on eight patients with nonseminomatous cancer in which cytoreductive surgery was associated with an apparent exacerbation of disease as determined both clinically and by serum marker levels. In some cases, cytoreductive surgery was followed by a dramatic rise in markers highly suggestive of a causal relationship. The mechanism to explain this does not exist as yet if in truth it is a real phenomenon. Further collaborative experience from other centers will have to be received before this can be accepted.

Ansari et al. [4] have studied the prognostic factors for the development of renal toxicity in 125 patients receiving cisplatin in combination regimens. The dosage of cisplatin was 20 mg/m^2 daily for 5 days 3 weeks for a minimum of 3–4 courses. No hydration was given to 47 patients. The remaining patients all received hydration with normal saline 100 cm^3/h beginning 12 h prior to the cisplatin dose, and continuing during drug treatment. No mannitol or furosemide were given. In this analysis, renal failure was defined as a serum creatinine in excess of 3.0 mg%. Sixteen cases of renal failure were observed and six of these patients died as a result. The correlation of renal failure development with prognostic factors reveals that concommitant administration of aminoglycoside antibiotics and hydration are significant variables. In 11 patients who both received aminoglycosides and did not receive hydration renal failure was noted in eight (71%). In the corresponding group, with hydration but without aminoglycosides, renal failure was observed in only 2 of 75 patients (3%) with the difference being highly significant ($p > 0.001$).

At the University of Minnesota [104] Raynaud's phenomena has been reported as a side-effect caused by PVB therapy for testicular cancer. They have reported on 38 patients treated with this regimen. They give Velban (0.15−0.2 mg/kg on days 1 and 2), bleomycin 30 units on days 2, 9, and 16, and cisplatin 20 mg/m^2 daily for 5 days. Velban alone is used for maintenance. Raynaud's phenomena was defined as well-demarcated blanching or cyanosis of the fingers on exposure to cold with reactive hyperemia on rewarming. This was found in 13 of the 38 patients. Two patients had single digital involvement and 11 had multiple digit involvement. Two patients developed trophic changes of the finger tips. The median duration of symptoms was 16 months with a gradual resolution after therapy was stopped. The syndrome could not be related to the total doses of any of the three drugs.

Preliminary studies from Britain [69] indicate that the PVB regimen has a significant impact on gonadal function. Twelve patients were studied who had no previous surgery to the paraaortic lymph nodes 3−18 months after receiving PVB therapy. All patients tested had an absence of motile sperm in their semen. In 71%, an increase in follicle-stimulating hormone (FSH) and luteinizing hormone (LH) was noted and all patients had one or the other of these hormones elevated. Biopsy of the normal remaining testicle in one patient showed grossly abnormal tubules with absence of spermatogenesis but marked Leydig's cell hypertrophy.

A variety of other combinations have been evaluated but none have been found superior to VB-3, PVB, or the VAB combinations. Einhorn and Donahue [30] briefly studied a combination of Adriamycin, bleomycin, and vincristine prior to initiating the PVB combination. The Adriamycin was administered at a dose of 75 mg/m^2 every 3 weeks while the vincristine was given at a dose of 1 mg followed in 6 h by 30 units of bleomycin intravenously. These latter two drugs were given weekly for 12 weeks. Eight patients were treated with this regimen from July 1973 through July 1974. There were three CRs and four PRs. The three complete remitting still remain disease-free although one of them relapsed after 7 months and was reinduced with PVB. One of the other complete responders was a pure choriocarcinoma who was disease-free at $4\frac{1}{2}$ years at the time of the literature report.

Jacobs and Muggia [42] in a recent review report on some additional combinations reported that the two drug combination of platinum and Adriamycin achieved three CRs of 18 patients with a 61% overall response rate. The duo of platinum plus bleomycin gave no complete responders in 14 cases but 79% achieved a PR.

The Toronto Testicular Tumor Study Group [98] uses a five drug induction regimen as follows: Cyclophosphamide 500 mg/m^2 IV day 1; vinblastine 5 mg/m^2 IV day 1; actinomycin D 1 mg/m^2 IV day 1; bleomycin 30 units IV push day 1 + 20 units/m^2 for 5 days by continuous infusion; cisplatin 120 mg/m^2 IV day 6. These courses are repeated monthly. Those patients who achieve a CR after three cycles are given no maintenance treatment. Those with only PR receive either additional drug and/or surgery. A total of 37 patients without prior drug treatment have been treated and CR observed in 31 (84%). Of these, 29 have remained in a disease-free state for a median of 14 months with a range of 1−34 months. Only one patient has relapsed, while the second committed suicide. Complete response was equally achieved in the 19 patients who had received prior irradiation and in those who did not, although toxicity was somewhat more severe in the irradiated group. This study is still an early one but indicates that maintenance drug treatment may not be required.

Table 39. VP-16 alone and in combination for previously treated metastatic nonseminomatous testicular cancer

Regimen	No. evaluable patients	No. CR	% CR	No. PR	% CR+PR
VP-16 100 mg/m^2 Daily × 3−5 every 3 weeks	2	0		2	100
VP-16 as above Cisplatin 20 mg/m^2 1 day × 5 every 3 weeks × 3−4 courses Adriamycin 40−50 mg/m^2 every 3 weeks × 3−4 courses Bleomycin 30 units IV weekly × 12	17	6	35	9	88
VP-16 as above Cisplatin as above Bleomycin as above	8	4	50	4	100
Total	27	10	37	15	92

Second Line Chemotherapy

An important question is what can be effectively used after failing on a primary combination. There are early results that indicate that VP-16 may be an important drug in this situation.

The European Organisation of Research on the Treatment of Cancer (EORTC) [16] has performed a phase II study of oral VP-16 in previously treated nonseminomatous testicular cancer. A total of 33 patients were entered, nearly all of whom had received two prior combination chemotherapy treatments. In addition, 20 had received prior irradiation. No data on performance status were given. The VP-16 dose was 175 mg/m^2 daily for 3 consecutive days every week. In 28 evaluable patients, PRs were observed in five (18%) and minor regressions in an additional seven. The median duration of PR was 3 months with a range of 1.5−4.5 months. The dose-limiting toxicity was marrow suppression. A WBC count below 2,000/mm^3 was observed in 10 of patients 28 and in 7 of 26 it went below 1,000/mm^3. It is clear that VP-16 exhibited activity in this heavily pretreated group of patients.

Williams and Einhorn [116] has studied VP-16 in combination or alone for patients failing on initial combination regimens (Table 39). With VP-16 combined with cisplatin, Adriamycin, and bleomycin, the CR rate was 35% with an overall response of 88%. Four of the PRs were rendered free of disease by resection of residual tumor. Two had residual carcinoma and two mature teratomas. Therefore, a total of 58.8% (10/17) attained a disease-free status and eight of these cases are still relapse-free at a median of 5+ months with the range being 2+−13.5+ months.

With VP-16 combined only with cisplatin and bleomycin the overall response rate was 100% with 50% achieving a CR. One of the PRs underwent resection and a mature teratoma was found. All five of the disease-free patients remain so at ranges of 3.5+ to 14+ months.

The toxicity in this heavily pretreated group was severe. All patients had alopecia, nausea, and vomiting. The WBC nadir was 1,100 cells/mm^3 and the platelet nadir

60,000. Eight patients required hospitalization for leukopenia and fever and four had documented infection but no deaths occurred. Two patients developed symptomatic nonfatal bleomycin-induced pulmonary fibrosis and another developed abnormal liver function studies possibly related to VP-16.

Brain Metastases

Since germinal neoplasms have a major homogeneous spread potential a propensity for brain metastases exists. The CNS is a pharmacologic sanctuary which requires special therapeutic strategies. As treatment began to achieve long-term survival gains in childhood, leukemia and oat cell lung cancer relapses in the CNS became a significant problem, the potential for the same situation now exists for testicular germinal neoplasms.

Williams and Einhorn [117] have examined the problem in 139 patients treated between July 1973 and March 1978 at the University of Indiana. Brain metastases were observed in 21 of these patients (15%). Patients who had symptoms or signs of CNS involvement had prompt brain scans and frequently CT. Carefully selected patients with solitary lesions were considered for surgical resection and postoperative radiation therapy. Otherwise, whole brain irradiation was used.

The incidence was most common in yolk sac lesions (3/6) and in choriocarcinoma (4/13 = 30.8%). The incidence in embryonal lesions was 10.1% (7/69) while in teratocarcinoma it was 11.8% (4/34). In 18 seminomas it was found in two cases (18.2%).

In four of the 21 patients the CNS involvement was observed at the time of the original diagnosis. In the rest it developed as a complication while under treatment. The median interval from the initial diagnosis until the development of brain metastases was 18 months with a range of 0−9.5 years. Once the diagnosis of CNS disease was made, the median survival was only 1.5 months, indicating that this complication is a major cause of morbidity and mortality in treated germinal neoplasms.

Einhorn and his group are now using routine brain scans in patients they consider to be at high risk for the development of CNS disease. These are patients with choriocarcinoma, or yolk sac histologies, extensive prior therapy or massive disease. It is hoped that routine brain scans will allow discovery of CNS metastases at an earlier point of time prior to the development of signs and symptoms.

Perspectives on Chemotherapy Data

There is now ample evidence that metastatic testicular cancer is potentially curable with aggressive combination chemotherapy. The regimens used are toxic and should only be administered by trained oncologists within a therapeutic setting of ample supportive care. It would seem realistic to approach metastatic testicular cancer at least as aggressively as acute myelocytic leukemia, where the cure potential is less. Physicians who diagnose testicular cancer should be sure to consult with, or refer to, oncologic treatment centers, so as to give every patient the optimal chance for recovery.

Anderson et al. [3] have recently analyzed some of the prognostic variables for complete response to drug treatment, utilizing data from M.D. Anderson,

Table 40. Prognostic factors for chemotherapy response

Prognostic factor	No. of patients	No. CR	% CR
I. Histology	127	92	72.4
1. Embryonal with or without seminoma			
2. Teratocarcinoma	89	40	44.9
3. Choriocarcinoma	20	8	40.0
4. Extragonadal primary tumor	11	4	36.4
II. Tumor burden			
1. Nonbulky			
A. Gynecomostia or elevated HCG	5	5	100.0
B. Supraclavicular nodes	3	3	100.0
C. Less than five pulmonary metastases (less than 2 cm in diameter)	39	33	84.6
D. Above plus nonbulky nodes	32	24	75.0
2. Bulky			
A. > five pulmonary metastases (> 2 cm diameter)	40	22	55.0
B. Large retroperitoneal nodes	39	21	53.8
C. Visceral involvement	20	2	10.0

Table 41. Some unanswered questions in testicular cancer combination chemotherapy

1. Is vinblastine + bleomycin + platinum superior to vinblastine + bleomycin alone?
2. What is the optimal dose level of vinblastine?
3. Are bleomycin continuous infusions superior to IV push or IM schedules?
4. What is the optimal dose level and schedule of platinum?
5. What is gained by adding more drugs to vinblastine + bleomycin + platinum:
   a) Actinomycin D
   b) Actinomycin D + alkylating agent
   c) Actinomycin D. + alkylating agent + adriamycin
6. What is the value of maintenance therapy after attainment of CR?

Sloan-Kettering, University of Indiana, and Roswell Park (Table 40). Histology is a critical variable. The CR rate in embryonal carcinoma lesions, with or without seminoma elements, is 72.4%, as compared with only 44.9% in teratocarcinoma and 40% in choriocarcinoma. In extragonadal lesions, the CR rate was also low at 36.4%. Another important prognostic variable ist the tumor burden being treated. The CR rate was 84.6% (33/39) in patients with fever than five pulmonary metastases less than 2 cm in diameter. In those with more extensive pulmonary metastases the rate dropped to 55% (22/40).

A variety of critical questions about the newer combination chemotherapy of testicular cancer remain unanswered (Table 41). These relate to the drugs used and their schedule intensity and duration. At this time, no regimen can be recommended as clearly superior to all others. The three major drugs are vinblastine, bleomycin, and platinum. None of the regimens including actinomycin, with or without alkylating agents and Adriamycin, have dramatically higher response rates than those reported for regimens without these drugs. In fact, a trial comparing vinblastine plus bleomycin alone and with the addition of platinum has never been reported. With regard to vinblastine, the ideal dose level still remains questionable. It does appear from ongoing studies of Einhorn and his group that lower doses can give an equivalent CR rate in their VBP regimen. What still remains to be determined is whether survival will be as good with the lower doses and whether better-risk patients are now being treated. Both the M.D. Anderson and the Sloan-Kettering groups feel that continuous infusions of bleomycin are superior to the earlier usage of the drug by IV push. Again, this can only be supported by historical controls and has to be measured against Einhorn's results without bleomycin infusions. Platinum is utilized on a range of schedules and dose levels, none of which can be established as definitive.

Adjuvant Chemotherapy

Testicular cancer raises some crucial questions about the adjuvant chemotherapy strategy. In testicular cancer, curative chemotherapy is available when patients develop metastatic relapse after their initial local and regional control chemotherapy. In such a situation, the need for adjuvant chemotherapy becomes less urgent. Adjuvant chemotherapy will potentially increase the cure rate when added to the local control modalities of surgery and irradiation. It will do so, however, at the cost of treating some patients with drugs unnecessarily. What has to be compared in a clinical research setting is the cure rate of two therapeutic approaches. The first involves optimal treatment with surgery and/or irradiation followed by close observation. At the earliest sign of metastatic relapse, curative intent chemotherapy should be used. In addition, surgical resection of isolated pulmonary metastases could be undertaken as indicated. The second approach would involve initial adjuvant chemotherapy and secondary salvage chemotherapy in those patients who relapse. Surgical resection of metastases could still be used as appropriate. A cost-benefit-ratio analysis will have to be made in comparing the two approaches. The benefit will be the overall cure rate. The cost will be the morbidity and mortality of therapy. It is important to realize that comparing the relapse-free survival of surgery against that obtained with surgery plus adjuvant chemotherapy will not be the crucial endpoint for analysis. It is conceivable that adjuvant chemotherapy will give a superior initial relapse-free survival rate but not be superior in terms of overall survival. In patients with stage II disease, at least half will be cured by their initial surgery. They will be receiving the costs of adjuvant chemotherapy without benefit. These costs involve not only the risks of physical morbidity and treatment mortality, but a range of psychosocial and economic costs, which must be considered as well.

The analysis of adjuvant drug trials in testicular cancer will, therefore, be a complex one involving ia range of different endpoints and cost-benefit analysis. An initial endpoint will be overall survival versus acute toxicity. The ultimate endpoint will be overall survival versus the acute and chronic toxicities of the treatment. These chronic toxicities will involve such aspects as long-term renal function and auditory function after cisplatin, neurologic function after vinca alkaloids, pulmonary function after

Table 42. Mini-VAB regimen for adjuvant chemotherapy in good-risk stage-II disease

Vinblastine	0.06 mg/kg	
Actinomycin D	0.02 mg/kg	} Weekly × 6
Bleomycin	0.25 mg/kg	
	↓	
	2-week interval	
Actinomycin D	0.02 mg/kg	
Chlorambucil	0.1 mg/kg 1 day × 7	} Every 14 days for 1 year
	↓	
Actinomycin D	0.02 mg/kg	
Chlorambucil	0.01 mg/kg	} Every 21 days for 1 year

bleomycin, and cardiac function after Adriamycin. In addition, the incidence of second malignancies possibly due to treatment will need to be carefully monitored. It will be tempting, after early analysis of adjuvant trials in testicular cancer, to report positive results based on initial relapse-free survival. This temptation should be tempered by the realization that early actuarial analysis can be overoptimistic and that successful secondary salvage may change the final picture dramatically.

At Sloan-Kettering [105], a modified, less toxic version of VAB I (Table 42) was administered to 62 patients with stage II disease who had undergone lymphadnectomy and had not received prior radiation. To date, 84% of the patients still remain disease-free. The most potent prognostic variable was found to be the extent of retroperitoneal lymph-node involvement. In 29 patients with bulky nodal disease or direct extranodal extension, relapses occurred in ten (35%) after VAB I adjuvant treatment, after a median follow-up of 25+ months. Nine of these ten relapses occurred within 8 months of lymphadnectomy. In 33 patients with only microscopic involvement of the nodes, none have relapsed, with a median follow-up of 19+ months. The features that make for good prognosis stage II in the Sloan-Kettering experience are ≤ five involved lymph nodes, none larger than 2 cm in diameter, no direct extralymphatic extension, and negative tumor markers after lymphadnectomy.

The VAB I experience has shown that a strategic split was indicated for stage II patients. Those with good prognostic features could continue on the modified VAB I regimen, but those without those features required more aggressive adjuvant chemotherapy. Therefore, 22 stage II patients with poor prognostic signs were then given the more aggressive VAB II regimen after lymphadnectomy. All 22 patients have remained disease-free for a median duration of 10+ months (Table 43).

It has been estimated that patients with pathologically documented stage II disease after lymphadnectomy have a 40% relapse potential. The chemotherapy data available would indicate that in the 40% of patients who would relapse after lymphadnectomy, about 60%−80% could be expected to achieve CR with drugs, with 60% of the entire group showing long-term disease-free survival indicative of cure. Thus, surgery with delayed chemotherapy at the time of relapse could be expected to salvage 85% of all patients (60% initially plus 25% at relapse) (Table 44). To show a 10% improvement with surgery plus immediate adjuvant chemotherapy would require 210 patients in a clinical trial. Even if this 10% improvement in cure rate were obtained, it would be necessary to weigh this against the cost of 60% receiving the risks of the drug

Table 43. Adjuvant chemotherapy after lymphadenectomy for stage II disease at Memorial Sloan-Kettering Cancer Center

	Regimens		
	Good prognostic features[a]	Poor prognostic features	
	VAB I	VAB I	VAB II
Number of patients	33	29	22
Number relapsed	0	10	0
Median follow-up time	19+	25+	10+

[a] ≤ five involved lymph nodes none longer than 2 cm; no extralymphatic extension; negative markers

Table 44. A perspective on adjuvant chemotherapy of testicular cancer expected salvage rate for sequential surgery and drugs in stage II testicular carcinoma

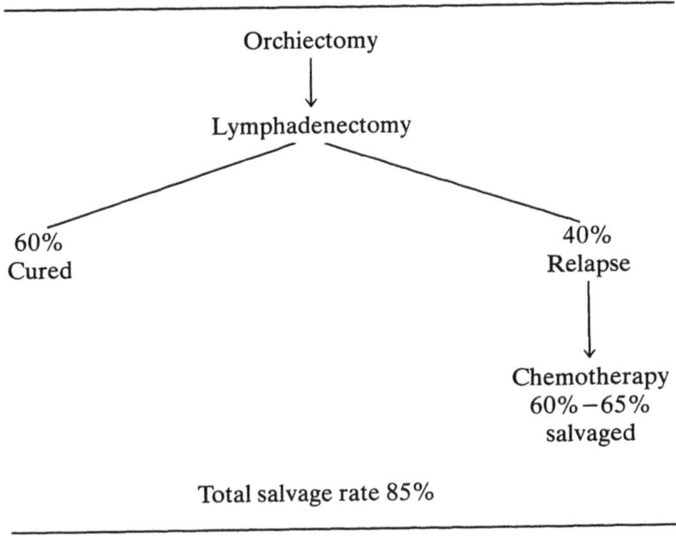

unnecessarily. Currently, a national study has been set up in the United States in which many of the major cooperative groups will participate and pool their patients. In this study, adjuvant chemotherapy in stage II with resectable lymph nodes will be compared to an initial therapeutic approach which eradicates all known disease (surgery), followed by monthly observation of the patient and the institution of potentially curative chemotherapy in those patients who develop recurrence. Excluded from this study will be patients whose markers remain abnormal 4 weeks after lymph node resection and those whose retroperitoneal nodes are clinically or surgically unresectable. The groups participating in this study will have a choice of two chemotherapy regimens. One is a modified PVB regimen and the other is a modified VAB III regimen (Table 45). As can be seen, these two regimens overlap in the usage of vinblastine, bleomycin, and platinum, but the dosage schedules differ significantly.

Table 45. Two adjuvant regimens utilized in the testicular cancer intergroup study

Vinblastine	− 15 mg/kg IV days 1 and 2 every 4 weeks for 8 weeks	4 mg/m^2 day 1 and 29
Bleomycin	30 units (total weekly dose) IV weekly for 8 consecutive weeks	30 mg IV push then mg/m^2/24-h infusion 6 days repeated every 28 days
Platinum	20 mg/m^2 daily for 5 days once every 4 weeks for two courses	120 mg/m^2 days 7
Actinomycin D Cyclophosphamide	−	1 mg/m^2 days 1 and 2 600 mg/m^2 days 1 and 2

In addition, the VAB adds actinomycin D and cyclophosphamide. In both approaches, only two cycles of adjuvant chemotherapy are given.

When relapse occurs in either of two protocol arms, four cycles of the same regimen used as adjuvant are to be administered. In the group that has received two adjuvant cycles the reinduction is modified to the amount of bleomycin and in the PVB arm the dose of vinblastine is lowered to 0.3 mg/kg every 4 weeks.

Peckham et al. [72] have reported a complex combined modality approach to malignant teratomas using the British classification. Patients included were those with abdominal nodes on lymphangiogram larger than 2 cm in maximum diameter or involvement of supradiaphragmatic and infradiaphragmatic lymph nodes without extralymphatic metastases. Included as well were patients with estralymphatic metastases. These patients were treated with vinblastine 15 mg/m^2 on days 1 and 2 and bleomycin 30 mg/day by continuous infusion over 24 h days 1−5. They received up to six courses at intervals of 4−5 weeks. After chemotherapy, selected patients proceeded to radiotherapy and in some cases surgery. A total of 56 patients were treated with 27 (48.2%) being alive and disease-free at the time of the report. It is difficult to evaluate this data in a comparative sense, since only some patients had measurable disease and no response figures are given. A separation is made into group I patients who had no extralymphatic metastases or less than three extralymphatic metastases and group II who were the rest with more extensive metastatic disease. In 33 group I patients, 23 (69.7%) were reported as alive and disease-free compared with 4 of 23 (17.4%) in group II. For previously untreated patients, the disease-free survival rates were 80.9% for group I and 16.7% for group II.

Rehabilitation

Since testicular cancer occurs predominantly in young men at the peak of their sexual activity and involves an organ related to fertility, a psychological impact is to be expected. The tumor can be viewed by patients as affecting sexual potency and masculinity despite the lack of any physiologic reason to support it. The emotional impact of this cancer has received surprisingly little attention despite this.

The psychological implications begin when a man first feels a scrotal mass. Delay in seeking medical attention may be due to fears, attitudes and emotions rather than ignorance that the mass could be a tumor. The patient, once he does seek attention, may seek to avoid orchiectomy at all costs and 'shop' around with a series of urologists thus losing valuable time in making the diagnosis. It is essential that the urologist make clear that an orchiectomy will not diminish potency, fertility, or virility.

The association of cancer of the genital organs and sex has been cloaked in folklore and myth for a long time. Speaking about it was a taboo for a long time thus leading to misconceptions and apprehensions on the part of many. Emotionally, some patients or their partners view genital cancers as punishment for some real or imagined sexual misconduct. As a result, there is shame, guilt, and fear particularly of transmitting the disease. This can all result in transient psychologically induced sexual dysfunction, diminished libido, and erectile difficulties. The physician must play a major role in dispelling the myths and reassuring the patient.

A common side effect of retroperitoneal lymphadnectomy is ejaculation without emission without loss of erectile and orgasmic activity. Infertility will result however. It is critically important that the patient understand that, while fertility will be lost, normal libido and orgasm will not. This loss of seminal emission is due to the interruption of the sympathetic ganglia at the L_2L_4 level since they are in close proximity to the involved nodes.

Radiotherapy to the abdomen in testicular cancer causes no change in sexual performance or drive though semen volume is diminished in one-third of patients. With shielding of the unaffected testicle during irradiation neither sexual performance nor fertility are impaired.

The modern successful combination chemotherapy regimens cause a great deal of toxicity and require a high level of patient commitment for a long period of time. Hospitalization is often required with a significant dislocation of work and personal life. Emotional support is an important component in achieving the patient compliance that offers the optimal potential for the attainment of cure.

Gorzynski et al. [36] report that anxiety tends to increase near the end of treatment with the patient expressing fears concerning the cessation of therapy. Such fears are transmitted by an increased number of telephone calls, outpatient visits, and complaints of nondescript symptoms.

References

1. Abelev GI (1971) Alpha-protein in oncogenesis and its association with malignant tumors. Adv Cancer Res 14: 295−358
2. Allaire F, Thieme E, Korst D (1961) Cancer chemotherapy with 5-fluorouracil alone and in combination with x-ray therapy. Cancer Chemother Rep 14: 59−75
3. Anderson T, Waldmann TA, Javadpour N, Glatstein E (1979) Testicular germ cell neoplasms: Recent advances in diagnosis and therapy. Ann Intern Med 90: 373−386
4. Ansari RH, Einhorn LH, Williams SD, Bond WH (1980) Short and long term platinum nephrotoxicity in patients with testicular cancer. PAACR-ASCO 21: 135
5. Astrakhan V, Monul F (1976) Combined chemotherapy of testicular tumors resistant to sarcolysin. Vopr Onkol 13: 87−90
6. Barski AA (1973) Diagnosis, staging and natural history of testicular tumors. Cancer 32: 1202−1205
7. Batata MA Chu FCH, Hilaris BS, Whitmore WF, Grabstald H, Golbey R (1980) TNM staging of testis cancer. Int J Radiat Oncol Biol Phys 6: 291−295

8. Batterman JJ, Delemarre JFM, Hart AAM, van Slooten EA, Tierie AH (1973) Testicular tumors: A retrospective study. Arch Chir Neere 25: 457–469
9. Benjamin RS, Wiernick PH, Bachur NR (1973) Adriamycin – efficacy, safety and pharmacological basis of a single dose schedule. Cancer Chemother Rep 57: 98
10. Blum RH, Carter SK, Agre K (1973) A clinical review of bleomycin – A new actineoplastic agent. Cancer 31: 903–914
11. Boctor ZN, Kurohara SS, Badib AO (1969) Current results from therapy of testicular tumors. Cancer 24: 8705
12. Boden G, Gibb R (1951) Radiotherapy and testicular neoplasms. Lancet 2: 1195–1197
13. Bradfield JS, Hagen RO, Yterdal DO (1973) Carcinoma of the testis: An analysis of 104 patients with germinal tumors of the testis other than seminoma. Cancer 31: 633–640
14. Buck, AS, Schamber DT, Maier JG, Lewis EL (1972) Supraclavicular node biopsy and malignant testicular tumors. J Urol 107: 619–621
15. Burney BT, Klatte EC (1980) Abdominal ultrasound and computed tomography in testicular cancer. In: Einhorn LH (ed) Testicular tumors, Masson, New York, p 83
16. Cavalli F, Klepp O, Renard J, Hansen HH, Alberto P (1980) A phase II study of oral VP-16 in patients with non-seminomatuus testicular cancer. PAACR-ASCO 21: 137
17. Chebotareva L (1964) Late results of sarcolysin therapy in tumors of the testes. Acta UN Int Congr Cancer II: 380
18. Cheng E, Cvitkovic E, Wittes RE, Golbey RB (1968) Germ cell tumors (II) VAB II in metastatic testicular cancer. Cancer 42: 2162–2168
19. Collins DM, Pugh RCB (1964) Classification and frequency of testicular tumors. Br J Urol [Suppl] 36: 1–11
20. Costa G, Hreshchyshyn MM, Holland JF (1962) Initial clinical studies with vincristine. Cancer Chemother Rep 24: 39–44
21. Cutler SJ, Young JL, Jr (eds) (1975) Third National Cancer Survey: Incidence data. Natl Cancer Inst Monogr 41
22. Devega SS, Silverman DT (1978) Cancer incidence and mortality trends in the United States 1935–1974. J Natl Cancer Inst 60: 545–571
23. Dixon FJ, Moore RA (1952) Tumors of the male sex organs. In: Atlas of tumor pathology, vol 8, fasc 316, 32. Armed Forces Institute of Pathology, Washington DC, pp 48–127 .
24. Donohue RE, Pfister RR, Weigel JW, Stonington OG (1977) Supraclavicular node biopsy in testicular tumors. Urology 9: 546–549
25. Dunnick NR (1979) Radiologic diagnosis in urologic cancer. In: Javadpour N (ed) Principles and management of urologic cancer. Williams and Williams, Baltimore, pp 127–167
26. Earle JE, Bagshaw MA, Kaplan HA (1971) Supervoltage radiation therapy of the testicular tumors. Am J Roentgerol Rad Ther Nucl Med 117: 653–661
27. Einhorn LH (1978) Combination chemotherapy with cis-diammine dichloroplatinum, vinblastine and bleomycin in disseminated testicular cancer: An update. In: Carter SK, Crooke ST, Umezawa H (eds) Bleomycin: Current Status and New Developments Academic, New York
28. Einhorn LH (1980) The role of surgery in disseminated testicular cancer. PAACR-ASCO 21: 159
29. Einhorn LH, Donahue JP (1977) Combination chemotherapy with cis-diammine dichloroplatinum, vinblastine and bleomycin in disseminated testicular cancer. Ann Intern Med 87: 293–298
30. Einhorn LH, Donahue JP (1979) Combination chemotherapy in disseminated testicular cancer: the Indiana University experience. Semin Oncol 6: 87–93
31. Einhorn LH, Williams SD (1980) The management of disseminated testicular cancer In: Einhorn LH (ed) Testicular tumors management and treatment. Masson, New York, pp 117–150

32. Ferber B, Handy VH, Gerhardt PR, Solomon J (1962) Cancer in New York state exclusive of New York City, 1941–1960. Albany, New York, Bureau of Cancer Control, New York State Department of Health
33. Friedman M (1950) Tumors of the testis and their treatment. In: Portman UV (ed) Clinical therapeutic radiology. Nelson, New York
34. Gitlin A, Boesman M (1967) Sites of serum alpha-fetoprotein synthesis in the human and in the rat. J Clin Invest 46: 1010–1016
35. Golbey RB, Reynolds TF, Vurgrin D (1979) Chemotherapy of metastatic germ cell tumors. Semin Oncol 6: 82–87
36. Gorzynski JG, Holland JC (1979) Psychological aspects of testicular cancer. Semin Oncol 6: 1
37. Hayes D, Cvitkovic E, Golbey B, Scheiner E, Krakoff IH (1976) Amelioration of renal toxicity of high dose cis-platinum diammine dichloride (CPPD) by Mannitol-induced diuresis. PAACR-ASCO 17: 169
38. Higby DJ, Wallace HJ, Albert D, Holland JF (1974) Diamminodichloroplatinum in the chemotherapy of testicular tumors. J Urol 112: 100–104
39. Hyman GA, Ultmann JE, Habif DV (1962) Factors to be considered in the clinical evaluation of a new chemotherapeutic agent (5-fluorouracil). Cancer Chemother Rep 16: 397–399
40. Jacobs EM (1970) Combination chemotherapy of metastatic testicular germinal cell tumors and soft part sarcomas. Cancer 25: 324–332
41. Jacobs EM, Johnson D, Wood DA (1966) Stage III metastatic malignant testicular tumors. Treatment with intermittent and combined chemotherapy. Cancer 19: 1697–1704
42. Jacobs EM, Muggia FM (1980) Testicular cancer: risk factors and the role of adjuvant chemotherapy. Cancer 45: 1782–1790
43. Javadpour N (1979) The value of biologic markers in diagnosis and treatment of testicular cancer. Semin Oncol 6: 37–47
44. Kennedy B (1969) Mithramycin treatment in testicular neoplasms. Am Soc Clin Oncol Abstr 20
45. Kohn J (1979) The value of apparent half-life assay of alpha-fetoprotein in the management of testicular teratoma. In: Lehmann FG (ed) Carcino-embryonic proteins: chemistry, biology, clinical applications, vol. II. New York, pp 383–386
46. Krikorian J, Daniels JR Brown BW, Hu SJ (1978) Variables for predicting serious toxicity (vinblastine dose, performance status and prior therapeutic experience): Chemotherapy for metastatic testicular cancer with cis-dichlorodiammine platinum (II), vinblastine and bleomycin. Cancer Treat Rep 62: 1455–1465
47. Lange PH, Hekmat K, Bosi G, Kennedy BJ, Fraky EE (1980) Accelerated growth of testicular cancer after cytoreductive surgery. Cancer 45: 1498–1506
48. Li FR, Fraumeni JF (1972) Testicular cancers in children: epidemiologic characteristics. J Natl Cancer Inst 48: 1575–1582
49. Li MC (1966) Management of choriocarcinoma and related tumors of uterus and testis. Med Clin North 45: 661
50. Li MC, Whitmore WF, Golbey R, Grabstald H (1960) Effects of combined drug therapy on metastatic cancer of the testis. J Am Med Assoc 174: 1291–1299
51. Lien HH, Kolbenstuedt A (1977) Phlebography, urography and lymphography in the diagnosis of metastatis from testicular tumors. Acta Radiol [Diagn] (Stockh) 18: 177–185
52. Lynch DF, Richie JO (1980) Supraclavicular node biopsy in staging testis tumor. J Urol 123: 39–40
53. Mackenzie A (1966) Chemotherapy of metastatic testic cancer: Results in 154 patients. Cancer 19: 1369–1376
54. Mackenzie AR, Duruman N, Whitmore WF (1967) Mithramycin in metastatic urogenital cancer J Urol 98: 116–119
55. Maier JG, Mittemeyer B (1977) Carcinomas of the testis. Cancer 39: 981–986

56. Maier JG, Sulak MH (1973) Radiation therapy in malignant testis tumors. Part II Carcinoma. Cancer 32: 1217−1226
57. McKay EN, Sellers HH (1966) A statistical review of malignant testicular tumors based on the experience of the Ontario Cancer Foundation Clinics, 1938 to 1961. Can Med Assoc J 94: 889−899
58. Mendelson D (1969) Combination chemotherapy of disseminated testicular Tumors. Proc Am Soc Clin Oncol Abstr 27
59. Merrin C (1976) A new method to prevent toxicity with high doses of cis-diammine platinum. PAACR-ASCO 17: 243
60. Monfardini S, Bajetta E, Musumeci R, Bonadonna G (1972) Clinical use of adriamycin in advanced testicular cancer. J Urol 108: 293−296
61. Moore C (1968) Triple chemotherapy in treatment of metastatic testicular neoplasms. J Urol 100: 527−529
62. Morrison AS (1975) Some social and medical characteristics of army men with testicular cancer. Am J Epidemiol 104: 511−516
63. Morrison AS (1976) Cryptorchidism, hernia, and cancer of the testis. J Natl Cancer Inst 56: 731−733
64. Mostofi FK (1979) Comparison of various clinical and pathological classifications of tumors of the testes. Semin Oncol 6: 26−30
65. Murphy WT (1967) Radiation therapy. Saunders, Philadelphia, pp 810−827
66. Nishi S (1970) Isolation and characterization of human fetal cypha-globulin from the sera of fetuses and a hepatoma patient. Cancer Res 30: 2507−2513
67. Nitschke R, Sterling K, Land V, Komp D (1976) Cis-platinum in childhood malignancies. PAACR-ASCO 17: 310
68. O'Bryan RM, Luce JK, Talley RW, Gottlieb JA, Bakel LH, Bonadonna G (1973) Phase II evaluation of adriamycin in human neoplasia. Cancer 32: 1−8
69. Oliver RTD, Wrigley PFM, Malpas JS (1980) Gonadal function after bleomycin, vinblastine and cisplatinum therapy. PAACR-ASCO 21: 426
70. Osieka R, Bruntsen U, Gallmeier WM (1976) Cis-diamminodichloroplatin (II) in der Behandlung therapieresistenter maligner Hodenteratome. Dtsch Med Wochenschr 101: 191−195
71. Peckham MJ, McElwain TJ (1974) Radiotherapy of testicular tumors. Proc R Soc Med 67: 400−404
72. Peckham MJ, McElwain TJ, Barret A, Hendry WF (1979) Combined management of malignant teratoma of the testis. Lancet II: 267−270
73. Percarpio B, Clements JC, McLeod DG, Sorgen SD, Cardinale FS (1979) Anaplastic semnoma − An analysis of 77 patients. Cancer 43: 2510−2513
74. Petersen GR, Lee JAH (1972) Secular trends of malignant tumors of the testis in white males. J Natl Cancer Inst 49: 339−354
75. Pitts N (1970) Clinical data accumulated by Pfizer for NDA for mithramycin. In: Carter SK, Friedman MA (eds) Proceedings of the chemotherapy conference on mithramycin: development and application. Cancer Therapy Evaluation Program, NCI, Bethesda, pp 33−44
76. Ream NW, Perlia CP, Wolter J, Taylor SG (1968) Mithramycin therapy in disseminated germinal testicular cancer. JAMA 204: 1030−1036
77. Rozencweig M, von Hoff DD, Slavik M, Muggia FM (1977) Cis-diamminodichloroplatinum (II) A new anticancer drug. Ann Intern Med 86: 803−812
78. Samson MK, Stephen RL, Rivkin S, Opipari M, Maloney T, Groppe CW, Fisher R (1979) Vinblastine, bleomycin and cis-dichlorodiammineplatinum (II) in disseminated testicular cancer: preliminary. Cancer Treat Rep 63: 1663−1667
79. Samuels ML, Howe CD (1970) Vinblastine in the management of testicular cancer. Cancer 25: 1009−1017
80. Samuels ML, Johnson DE, Holoye PY (1975) Continuous intravenous bleomycin therapy with vinblastine in stage III testicular neoplasia. Cancer Chemother Rep 59: 563−570

81. Samuels ML, Lanzotti VJ, Holoye PY, Boyle LE, Smith TL, Johnson DE (1976) Combination chemotherapy in germinal cell tumors. Cancer Treat Rev 3: 185–204
82. Samuels ML, Johnson DE, Brown B (1979) Velban plus continuous infusion bleomycin (VB-3) in stage III advanced testicular cancer. In: Johnson DE, Samuels ML (eds) Cancer of the Genitourinary Tract. Raven, New York, p 159
83. Scardino PT, Cox HA, Waldmann TA (1977) The value of serum tumor markers in the staging and prognisis of germ cell tumors of the testis. J Urol 118: 994–999
84. Schaner EG, Chang AE, Doppman ML, Conkle DM, Flye MW, Rosenberg SA (1978) Comparison of computed and conventional whole lung tomography in detecting pulmonary nodules. AJR 131: 51–54
85. Shaw RK, Bruner JA (1964) Clinical evaluation of vincristine. Cancer Chemother Rep 42: 45–48
86. Silvay O, Yagoda A, Wittes R, Whitmore W, Golbey R (1973) Treatment of germ cell carcinomas with a combination of actinomycin D, vinblastine and bleomycin. PAACR-ASCO 14: 68
87. Skinner DG (1977) Advances in the management of non-seminomatous germinal tumors of the testis. Br J Urol 49: 553–560
88. Smart CR, Rochlin DB, Nah-M AM, Silva A, Wagner LD (1961) Clinical experience with vinblastine sulfate in squamous cell carcinoma and other malignancies. Cancer Chemother Rep 34: 31–45
89. Smithers DW, Wallace ENK (1962) Radiotherapy in the treatment of patients with seminomas and teratomas of the testicle. Br J Urol 34: 422–435
90. Snyder W, Rodensky P, Lieberman B (1964) Regression, relapse and regression of metastatic seminoma by cyclophosphamide. Cancer Chemother Rep 41: 34–40
91. Sogani PC, Vugrin D, Whitmore WF, Bains M, Herr H, Golbey R (1980) Experience with combination chemotherapy and surgery in the management of advanced germ cell tumors. PAACR-ASCO 21: 401
92. Solomon J, Steinfeld JL, Batemen JR (1967) Chemotherapy of germinal tumors. Cancer 20: 747–750
93. Spigel SC, Coltman CA (1974) Vinblastine and bleomycin therapy for disseminated testicular tumors. Cancer Chemother Rep 58: 213–216
94. Spigel SC, Stephens RL, Haas CD (1978) Chemotherapy of disseminated germinal tumors of the testis – comparison of vinblastine and bleomycin with vincristine, bleomycin and actinomycin D. Cancer Treat Rep 62: 129–130
95. Staubitz WJ, Early KS, Magoss IV, Murphy GP (1973) Surgical management of non-seminomatous germinal tumors. Cancer 32: 1200–1211
96. Staubitz WJ, Magoss IV, Grace JT, Schenk WG (1969) Surgical management of testis tumors. J Urol 101: 350–355
97. Steinfeld JL, Solomon J, Marsh AA, Hazen JG, Bateman JR (1966) Chemical therapy of patients with advanced metastatic germinal tumors. J Urol 96: 933–940
98. Sturgeon JFG, Alison RE, Comisarow RH, Bergsagei DE (1980) Advanced non-seminomatous testicular tumors: maintenance chemotherapy is unnecessary. PAACR-ASCO 21: 153
99. Sulak MH (1970) Classification of different pathologic types. J Am Med Assoc 213: 91–93
100. Tan C, Etcubanas E, Wollner N et al. (1973) Adriamycin, an antitumor antibiotic in the treatment of neoplastic disease. Cancer 32: 9–17
101. Tan CT, Golbey RB, Yab CL, Wollner N, Hackethal CA, Murphy LM, Dargeon HW, Burchenal JH (1960) Clinical experiences with acinomycins D, KS2 and F1 (KS4). Ann NY Acad Sci 898: 426–444
102. Vaitukaitus JL, Braunsten GD, Ross GT (1972) A radioimmunoassay which specifically measures human chorionic gonadotropin in the presence of human luteinizing hormone. Am J Obstet Gynecol 113: 751–758
103. van Derwerf-Messing B (1976) Radiotherapeutic treatment of testicular tumors. Int J Radiat Oncol Phys 1: 235–248

104. Vogelzang NJ, Bosl GJ, Johnson K, Kennedy BJ (1980) Raynauds phenomenon following induction chemotherapy for testicular tumor. PAACR-ASCO 21:151
105. Vugrin D, Cvitkovic E, Whitmore WF, Golbey RB (1979) Adjuvant chemotherapy in resected non-seminomatous germ cell tumors of the testis: Stages I-II. Semin Oncol 6:94–99
106. Vugrin D, Dukeman M, Whitmore W, Golbey R (1980) VAB-6: Progress in chemotherapy of germ cell tumors. PAACR-ASCO 21:426
107. Waldmann TA, McIntyre KR (1972) Serum alpha-fetoprotein levels in patients with ataxia-telengiectasia. Lancet 2:1112–1115
108. Wallace S, Jing B (1970) Lymphangiography: Diagnosis of nodal metastases form testicular malignancies. JAMA 213:94–96
109. Walsh PC, Kaufman JJ, Coulson WF, Goodwin WE (1971) Retroperitoneal lymphadnectomy for testicular tumors. JAMA 217:309–312
110. Whitelaw DM, Cowan DH, Cassidy EB, Patterson TA (1963) Clinical experience with vincristine. Cancer Chemother Rep 30:12–20
111. Whitmore W (1962) Some experience with retroperitoneal lymph node dissection and chemotherapy in the management of testis neoplasms. Br J Urol 34:436–447
112. Whitmore WF (1968) The treatment of germinal tumors of the testis. In: Cancer management. Lippencott, Philadelphia, p 347
113. Whitmore WF (1970) Germinal tumors of the testis. In: Proceedings of the sixth national cancer conference. Lippencott, Philadelphia, pp 219:245
114. Whitmore WF (1979) Surgical treatment of adult germ cell tumors. Semin Oncol 6:55–69
115. Williams SD, Einhorn LH (1980) Cisplatin chemotherapy of testicular cancer. In: Prestayko AW, Crooke ST, Carter SK (eds) Cisplatin current status and new developments. Academic, New York, pp 323–328
116. Williams SD, Einhorn LH (1980) VP-16-213: An active drug in germinal neoplasms. In: Einhorn LH (ed) Testicular tumors management and treatment. Masson, New York, pp 169–178
117. Williams SD, Einhorn LH (1980) Brain metastases in testicular cancer. In: Einhorn LH (ed) Testicular tumors management and treatment. Masson, New York, pp 179–184
118. Wilson W (1970) Chemotherapy of human solid tumors with 5-fluorouracil. Cancer 13:1230–1239
119. Wyatt JK, McAninch LN (1967) A chemotherapeutic approach to advanced testicular carcinoma. Can J Surg 10:421–426
120. Yarbro JW, Kennedy BJ (1967) A comparison of the rate of recovery from inhibition of RNA synthesis in mouse liver and transplantable glioma. Cancer Res 27:1779–1782

Treatment of Metastatic Renal Cell Carcinoma

F. M. Torti

Division of Medical Oncology, Stanford University Medical Center, Palo Alto, CA, USA

Renal cell carcinoma is the third most common urologic cancer. There are approximately 7,000 deaths annually due to this malignancy. In 1982, it is estimated that there will be 18,000 new cases identified. The disease is three times more common in males than females.

In order to discuss appropriately the management of metastatic renal cell carcinoma, there are certain general features of renal cell carcinoma that require brief discussion so as to place the treatment of metastatic disease in perspective. Four issues need to be addressed: (1) The natural history of renal cell carcinoma; (2) the adequate staging for renal cell carcinoma, particularly with regard to the appropriate use of angiography and computerized tomography (CT) scanning; (3) the impact of surgical technique on survival; (4) the role of radiation therapy in renal cell carcinoma.

Natural History

It is often forgotten that renal cell carcinoma, even when metastatic, is a disease with a natural history that is quite variable. Although most patients who have metastatic disease die within a few years, approximately 20% of patients live greater than three years with their metastatic disease [23]. In the series of patients with stage III and IV disease of Papac et al. [99], 25% lived up to 10 years, although median survival was 10 months. Factors that seem to influence survival once metastases have occurred include: (1) Time from nephrectomy to diagnosis of metastases; (2) recurrence or persistence of local tumor (some series); (3) site(s) of metastases. This occasionally prolonged survival with metastatic disease is not accounted for by the rare patients with spontaneous regression of metastatic disease, who are discussed later in the section. Equally important, the risk of recurrence is substantial even a number of years after presumed cure. McNichols et al. reported that of the 158 patients in their series who were alive and free of disease at 10 years, 18 (11%) recurred 10 years or longer after nephrectomy [81].

Staging

Appropriate pretherapeutic evaluation is necessary to define those patients in whom the attempt to cure with surgery would be appropriate. In addition to routine tests such as chest X-ray and liver function tests, preoperative evaluation should include inferior vena cavagram and CT scan of the kidney and adjacent retroperitoneal structures, and

Recent Results in Cancer Research. Vol. 85
© Springer-Verlag Berlin · Heidelberg 1983

Table 1. Staging of Renal Cell Carcinoma (from Robson)

Stage I.	Tumor confined to the kidney
Stage II.	Perirenal involvement but confined within Gerota's fascia
Stage III.	Regional invasion A. Renal vein or inferior vena cava involvement B. Lymphatic involvement C. Combination of A and B
Stage IV.	A. Involvement of adjacent organs other than the adrenals B. Distant metastases

possibly renal arteriography. Computerized tomography appears superior to angiography in terms of detection of local invasion through the capsule to surrounding structures [77]. Renal hilar nodes as well as paraaortic lymph nodes can also be detected by this technique. Inferior vena cavagram is superior, however, in the detection of caval extension of the tumor. Chest tomography should also be considered preoperatively as well. In one series of patients with negative chest X-ray results, 10% of patients were identified as having positive nodes upon whole-lung tomography [10].

Surgery

A radical nephrectomy, the removal of the entire kidney with Gerota's fascia intact, is the current standard treatment for renal carcinoma. Survival after radical nephrectomy appears to be significantly better than survival after simple nephrectomy in most, but not all, reported series: Robson et al. reported a 66% survival at 10 years with radical nephrectomy versus a 22% survival at 10 years with simple nephrectomy [107]. Others have not found such a wide differential in survival [117]. These are not randomized studies, however, and patient selection may play an important role in these differences. Whether a lymphadenectomy improves survival has been debated. Overall survival if lymph nodes are positive is < 20%, regardless of inclusion or extent of lymphadenectomy [24].
In addition, Robson and others have identified factors that affect the prognosis of renal cell carcinoma: 1) The extent of metastases; 2) histologic grade of tumor; 3) regional lymph node involvement; 4) involvement of the renal vein [15, 83, 107]. Pathologically, these are reflected in the staging of renal cell carcinoma first suggested by Robson which is still widely used (Table 1).

Radiotherapy

Primary radiation therapy as the sole modality treatment for renal cell carcinoma is a toxic and ineffective therapy. As an adjuvant to surgery, randomized clinical trials with both preoperative and postoperative radiation have shown no benefit on survival and cannot be routinely recommended [62]. Van der Werf-Messing studied 141 cases of renal cell carcinoma randomized to surgery alone versus preoperative radiation

therapy of 3,000 rad in 3 weeks. No survival advantage was seen. Local recurrence seemed to occur more frequently in the radiation therapy group, but this was thought to be an artifact of more careful surveillance [140].
Finney [31] studied 100 patients randomized to surgery versus surgery plus 5,500 rad in 5½ weeks postoperatively. Survival was again similar, and there was no appreciable impact on local recurrence.

Treatment of Metastatic Disease

There is a wide range of options, mostly ineffective, in the treatment of metastatic renal cell carcinoma. These include surgical removal of a single metastasis of renal cell carcinoma, surgical removal or infarction of the involved kidney in patients with metastatic disease in an attempt to affect the natural history of the metastatic disease, surgical removal of multiple metastases, hormonal therapy, and chemotherapy.

Surgical Removal of Single and Multiple Metastases

Perhaps the most successful treatment of metastatic disease is local excision of limited metastatic disease. A number of series suggest that about 25%–35% of patients have distant metastases at the time of diagnosis. Only 1%–3% of patients at presentation will have a single metastatic focus, however. With aggressive surgical treatment of these single foci of metastatic disease (usually lung), approximately 35% will be alive at 5 years [131]. Extension of this approach to selected patients with a few isolated foci of disease has been suggested [118]. Some series on surgical removal of metastatic foci report on excision of metastatic foci at the time of diagnosis of the primary tumor [131]. Asynchronous metastases, i.e., metastases that occur after a nephrectomy for localized disease, have been the subject of less detailed analysis. However, these metastases may confer a better prognosis if surgically removed than solitary metastases excised at initial diagnosis [95].

Nephrectomy to Control Metastatic Disease

In contrast to the relative effectiveness of surgery in the treatment of localized metastases, routine use of nephrectomy to influence the natural history of multiple metastatic foci has not been shown to be effective [23, 59], with the possible exception of isolated bone metastases [86].
Treatment of metastatic disease would not be complete without a discussion of spontaneous regression. This is a quite rare occurrence with Freed et al. [34] finding in their review of the literature only 48 cases with acceptable documentation of this event. In 1981, Fairlamb found documentation for 67 cases [27].
Many of these cases have had a nephrectomy which has led to the argument that nephrectomy induces spontaneous regression [37]. However, the rarity of spontaneous regression, compared to the quite frequent use of nephrectomy in this setting, makes this an unwarranted procedure. In addition, Freed et al. noted that in three of the reported cases of spontaneous regression, regression occurred without surgical

intervention; thus surgery is not a necessary concomitant of spontaneous regression.

Recently, infarction of the primary tumor followed by nephrectomy 4–7 days later has been utilized in patients with metastatic diseases [124]. This was followed by parenteral progestational therapy. Response rate of metastatic lesions has been high: 7 of 50 cases complete response (CR); 5 of 50 cases partial response (PR). However, not all studies of embolization have been positive [79]. These positive results will need to be confirmed and compared to conservative therapy before such an approach can be routinely adopted.

Other approaches that modulate the immune response have been utilized, including *Coryne bacterium parvum* [47], xenogeneic immune ribonucleic acid [106], and bacillus Calmette-Guerin (BCG) [90]. These approaches have often been coupled to nephrectomy and have generally had insufficient numbers of patients to demonstrate conclusively the value of the immune modulator.

Hormonal Treatment

The hormonal therapy of metastatic renal cell carcinoma is palliative in intent, marginal in effectiveness, and nearly universally utilized. The use of hormones in renal cell carcinoma has some rational basis in animal model systems. Estrogens induce renal tumors in some species [14]. Further, testosterone administration is associated with renal hypertrophy. However, a causal link between estrogen levels or duration of estrogen exposure in renal cell carcinoma has never been definitely established.

Bloom and Wallace first treated patients with renal cell carcinoma with hormonal therapy [12]. In 1971 and then in 1973 Bloom reported on a series of 80 patients plus a review of the literature [13, 14]. His conclusions set the basis for the widespread utilization of hormonal therapy in renal cell carcinomas. He concluded that objective tumor regressions were seen in 11 of 80 patients treated with progestational agents or testosterone. Responses usually occurred in 6 weeks after initiation of the treatment; men appeared to respond more frequently than women. Bloom noted that a different pattern of regression of the metastatic disease occurred with hormonal therapy when compared to spontaneous regressions of renal cell carcinoma; spontaneous regressions were almost always pulmonary, whereas hormonal regressions occurred at a variety of nonpulmonary sites as well. This different pattern of response supported their hypothesis that there was a different underlying mechanism for spontaneous and hormonal mediated regression.

Bloom's review of the literature suggested a 15% response rate (42 of 272 cases) of patients treated with hormonal agents, although it is often reported as higher. Definition of response both in his own series as well in the series he reviewed were quite variable. Many of these would not be accepted responses in modern chemotherapeutic trials. Subsequent to 1973, the number of series have shown very low response rates to progestational agents (Tables 2, 3). Hrushesky reported that of the 415 patients treated with hormonal agents between 1971 and 1976, only 2% responded [55].

Some series of hormonal therapies allow a 25% reduction in tumor size to be considered an objective response. Some series include stabilization of disease as an objective response. Some series include mixed responses (that is, one tumor nodule regression with others remaining stable as objective responses). Many series do not

Table 2. Progestational agents in renal cell carcinoma

Author (year)	No. of Patients	No. of CR & PR	MR or unspecified response	Stabilization	Subjective response	Reference no.
Melander (1967)	20	4	–	–	–	[82]
Alberto (1974)	17	0	0	0	0	[1]
Wagle (1971)	35	–	6	–	–	[134]
Morales (1975)	18	0	0	0	3	[89]
Bloom (1973)	80	–	11	–	45	[14]
Lokich (1975)	23	1	0	0	0	[76]
van der Werf-Messing (1971)	31	–	3	5	12	[142]
Peterson (1974)	14	2	0	1	6	[102]
Talley (1969)	16	2[a]	–	–	–	[126]
Talley (1973)	61	7	–	–	–	[125]
Paine (1970)	15	2	–	1	–	[96]
Samuels (1968)	23	3	–	–	–	[113]
Sadoff (1974)	16	–	3	–	–	[110]
Jenkin (1967)	6	0	0	0	–	[58]
Papac (1977)	12	0	–	–	–	[99]
Woodruff (1967)	4	1	–	–	–	[146]
Ramirez (1971)	27	0	–	–	–	[103]
Hahn (1979)	85	3	–	–	–	[45]
Stolbach (1981)	22	1	4	17	–	[121]

CR, complete response; PR, partial response: 50% reduction of the product of the tumor diameters; MR, minimal response: < 50% (often 'response' without any indication of magnitude of response); O, none; –, not recorded
[a] One 3 months after initiation of therapy and the other 9 months after initiation of therapy

Table 3. Androgen therapy in renal cell carcinoma

Author (year)	No. of Patients	No. of CR & PR	MR or unspecified response	Stabilization	Subjective response	Reference no.
Jenkin (1967)	15	1	–	2	7	[58]
Tally (1969)	11	0	0	0	0	[126]
Wagle (1971)	27	1	1	–	–	[134]
Lokisch (1975)	37	0	0	0	0	[76]
van der Werf-Messing (1971)	2	0	0	0	1	[142]
Paine (1970)	6	0	–	–	–	[96]
Talley (1973)	37	0	–	–	–	[125]
Alberto (1974)	23	0	–	–	–	[1]
Morales (1975)	20	1	–	3	0	[89]
Papac (1977)	17	1	1	2	–	[99]
Samuels (1968)	11	1	–	–	–	[113]

CR, complete response; PR, partial response: 50% reduction of the product of the tumor diameters; MR, minimal response: < 50% (often 'response' without any indication of magnitude of response); O, none; –, not recorded

Table 4. Antiestrogens in renal cell carcinoma

Drug Author (year)	No. treated	No. of CR & PR	MR/stabi- lization	Subjective response	Reference no.
Nafoxidine					
Paladine (1979)	10	3	–	–	[97]
Feun (1979)	21	1	7	–	[30]
Stolbach (1981)	19	3	4	–	[121]
Tamoxifen					
Weiselberg (1981)	9	0	0	–	[138]
Papac (1980)	3	0	–	–	[98]
Mulder (1979)	23	0	2	–	[91]
Glick (1980)	12	0	2	–	[38]
Legha (1976)	4	2	–	–	[72]
Al Saraff (1979, 1981)	79	2	14	–	[2, 3]
Ferrazzi (1980)	12	0	3	–	[29]
Tisman (1976)	4	0	2	–	[128]
Concolino (1978)	1	0	0	–	[19]

CR, complete response; *PR*, partial response: 50% reduction of the product of the tumor diameters; *MR*, minimal response: < 50% (often 'response' without any indication of magnitude of response); *O*, none; –, not recorded

specify any criteria for objective response. Tables 2 and 3 list the response rates in the literature, first for progestational agents and secondly for androgen treatment.

Some generalizations about hormonal treatment can be made in spite of the poor quality of data. It appears that most responses occur within 6 weeks of initiation of hormonal therapy and the prolonged utilization of hormonal therapy in the face of a nonresponse is not warranted. Responses seem to occur more frequently in men, although there are reported responses in females as well. The response rate seems higher for progestational agents than androgens, although this would be at best a tentative conclusion. There does not appear to be a clear dose-response relationship for progestational agents, although this has never been tested in a careful manner. Route (PO or IM), dose, and schedule appear to affect peak and steady-state serum levels of medroxyprogesterone acetate [80, 111]. However, the clinical correlations of these observations are lacking. Further, the subtype of progestional or androgenic agent utilized appears to have little demonstrable effect.

Antiestrogens have been reported to have activity in renal cell carcinoma. Both nafoxidine and tamoxifen have been studied, and minimal to modest activity has been reported for both agents (Table 4).

Hormone receptor assays, which have been useful in predicting responses in breast cancer, have thus far not proved helpful in predicting which patients will respond to any of the commonly used hormonal treatments in renal cell carcinoma.

Although there are a large number of studies that combine hormonal and chemotherapy, some of the highest response rates were recorded with presumably inactive chemotherapy, such as Adriamycin and vincristine [57].

Table 5. Trials of simultaneous hormonal and chemotherapy in renal cell carcinoma

Author (year)	Hormonal agent	Chemotherapeutic agents	No. of patients	No. of CR & PR	MR/stabi-lization	Subjective response	Reference no.
Hahn (1978)	MPA	CCNU	38	4	4	–	[43, 44]
Hahn (1978)	MPA	Vinblastine	38	8	5	–	[43, 44]
Levi (1980)	Tamoxifen	HDMTX, vinblastine, bleomycin	14	5	6	–	[75]
Ishmael (1980)	Depo-provera	Adriamycin, vincristine, BCG	38	18	–	–	[56]
Talley (1979)	MPA	Cyclophosphamide, vinblastine, prednisone, hydroxyurea	42	8	7	–	[127]
Katakkar (1978)	MPA	Adriamycin vinblastine, hydroxyurea	8	2	3	–	[63]
Voiska (1978)	Delalutin	CCNU, vinblastine	17	0	4	–	[133]
Richards (1977)	Methylprednisolone	CCNU, bleomycin	16	1	4	–	[105]
Richards (1977)	Methylprednisolone	CCNU, bleomycin, Adriamycin	14	3	5	–	[105]
Patel (1978)	Testosterone + MPA	Vincristine, actinomycin-D, cyclophosphamide	4	0	–	–	[101]
Swanson (1980)	Estramustine	Estramustine	11	0	7	–	[122, 123]
Dorn (1975)	MPA	Vinblastine	1	1	–	–	[26]

CR, complete response; *PR*, partial response: 50% reduction of the product of the tumor diameters; *MR*, minimal response: < 50% (often 'response' without any indication of magnitude of response); *O*, none; –, not recorded; *MPA*, medroxyprogesterone

Chemotherapy of Renal Cell Carcinoma

There is a general and near universal agreement on the marginal utility of chemotherapy in renal cell carcinoma. Surprisingly, however, a number of drugs have not been tested adequately in this relatively common tumor. Many of the series that have been collected include a large number of patients in phase I or early drug-oriented phase II trials of drugs with only one to five patients with renal cell carcinoma included. These studies could easily overlook significant activity due to both the patient population and the duration of therapy. Nevertheless, a number of reviews of this subject have been done. Woodruff et al. reviewed the literature in 1967 [146], Talley in 1973 [125], Carter and Wasserman in 1975 [17], and Hogan in 1979 [52]. The tables (below) detail the responses for chemotherapeutic agents. Moderate activity for vinblastine, minimal activity for the nitrosoureas, and essentially negative activity for the other drugs tested is evident.

Although vinblastine is frequently utilized in the treatment of renal cell carcinoma, and a dose-response effect has been noted [54, 92], it is surprising how few patients have been evaluated in phase II studies (Table 7). There are few studies with large patient numbers. One of the highest response rates is reported by Hagan et al. in 1974 [40]. However, the criteria of response are not outlined in that report. The response rate in the other large series, from the Eastern Cooperative Oncology Group, is modest (4 of 44 cases) [44]. Vincristine, vindestine, VM-26, and VP-16 have all shown minimal activity.

Table 6. Single agent chemotherapy: plant alkaloids

Drug Author (year)	No. of patients	No. of CR & PR	MR/stabi- lization	Subjective response	Reference no.
Vinblastine					
Hahn (1977)	10	0	3	–	[42]
Horn (1967)	2	1	–	–	[53]
Hagan (1974)	35	11	–	–	[40]
Hahn (1978)	44	4	–	3/44	[44]
Frei (1961)	3	0	–	–	[35]
Smart (1964)	2	0	–	1	[119]
Wright (1963)	(?)	0	0	3	[147]
Hill (1961)	5	1	2	–	[48]
Vincristine					
Horn (1967)	1	0	0	–	[53]
Costa (1962)	3	0	0	–	[20]
Vindestine					
Wong (1977)	17	0	6	–	[145]
VM-26					
Hire (1979)	12	0	–	–	[50]
VP-16					
Hahn (1979)	36	1	–	–	[45]

CR, complete response; PR, partial response: 50% reduction of the product of the tumor diameters; MR, minimal response: < 50% (often 'response' without any indication of magnitude of response); O, none; –, not recorded

Alkylating agents have been widely tested in renal cell carcinoma (Table 7). Cyclophosphamide, cis-platinum, chlorzotocin, and 1-(2-Chloroethyl)-3-(4-methylcyclohexyl)-1-nitrosourea (MeCCNU) have no or minimal activity. Thiotepa, chlorambucil, and 5-(3,3-Dimethyl-1-triazeno)imidazole-4-carboxamide (DTIC) have not been adequately studied (less than 15 patients). 1(2-Chloroethyl)-3-cyclohexyl-1-nitrosourea (CCNU) has a cumulative response rate of 16% (8 of 50 cases).

Table 7. Single agent chemotherapy: alkylators and nitrosoureas

Drug Author (year)	No. of patients	No. of CR & PR	MR/stabilization	Subjective response	Reference no.
Cyclophosphamide					
Solomon (1963)	1	0	0	–	[120]
Atkins (1962)	5	1	0	–	[7]
Anders (1961)	1	0	–	–	[4]
Fox (1965)	7	2	0	1	[33]
Bergsagel (1960)	2	1	–	–	[11]
Shnider (1960)	6	0	0	–	[116]
Dick (1961)	6	0	1	–	[25]
Wajsman (1980)	12	0	5	–	[135]
Kiruluta (1975)	10	0	0	0	[67]
Hahn (1979)	54	2	–	–	[45]
Chlorambucil					
Moore (1968)	14	2	5	–	[87]
Thiotepa					
·Hahn (1977)	7	1	1	–	[42]
Azetepa					
Choy (1967)	3	1	–	–	[18]
CCNU					
Hahn (1977)	7	0	1	–	[42]
Mittleman (1973)	20	4	2	–	[85]
Merrin (1975)	23	4	2	–	[83]
DTIC					
Luce (1970)	2	0	0	0	[78]
MeCCNU					
Hahn (1978)	45	2	8	–	[44]
Chlorzotocin					
Gralla (1979)	21	0	3	–	[39]
CIS-platinum					
Rodriguez (1978)	23	0	8	–	[109]
Phosphamide					
Fossa (1980)	11	1	1	–	[32]
Uracil mustard					
Schumacher (1963)	1	1	0	–	[115]

CR, complete response; *PR*, partial response: 50% reduction of the product of the tumor diameters; *MR*, minimal response: < 50% (often 'response' without any indication of magnitude of response); *O*, none; –, not recorded

The response rate to anthracycline and other antibiotics is reviewed in Table 8. Although these agents are generally thought of as inactive, the number of patients in which these drugs have been tested is quite small for most of these agents. Table 9 shows some of the results of folate antagonists. Some activity is demonstrated for methotrexate but numbers are quite small and require confirmation.

Table 8. Single-agent chemotherapy: antibiotics

Drug Author (year)	No. of patients	No. of CR & PR	MR/stabi- lization	Subjective response	Reference no.
Adriamycin					
O'Bryan (1973)	15	0	0	–	[94]
Mitomycin C					
Watne (1967)	1	1	0	–	[137]
Kato (1979) (microencapsulated)	2	1	1	2	[64]
Actinomycin					
Watne (1960)	4	0	0	–	[136]
Hahn (1981)	61	1	–	–	[46]
Bleomycin					
Johnson (1975)	15	2[a]	–	–	[61]
Hahn (1977)	7	0	2	–	[42]
Mithramycin					
Kofman (1963)	2	0	–	–	[71]

CR, complete response; PR, partial response: 50% reduction of the product of the tumor diameters; MR, minimal response: < 50% (often 'response' without any indication of magnitude of response); O, none; –, not recorded
[a] Mixed responses

Table 9. Single-agent chemotherapy: folate antagonists

Drug Author (year)	No. of patients	No. of CR & PR	MR/stabi- lization	Subjective response	Reference no.
Methotrexate					
Andrews (1967)	14	1	–	–	[5]
Baumgartner (1980)	8[a]	2	0	0	[8, 9]
Methodichlorophen					
Hindmarsh (1979)	10	3	–	–	[49]
Triazinate (Baker's antifol)					
Hahn (1981)	59	3	–	–	[46]
Bukowski (1980)	15	1	–	–	[16]

CR, complete response; PR, partial response: 50% reduction of the product of the tumor diameters; MR, minimal response: < 50% (often 'response' without any indication of magnitude of response); O, none; –, not recorded
[a] Citrovorum factor rescue

Table 10. Single-agent chemotherapy: purine and pyrimidine antagonists

Drug Author (year)	No. of patients	No. of CR & PR	MR/stabi- lization	Subjective response	Reference no.
5-fluorouracil					
Weiss (1961)	2	0	0	–	[139]
White (1962)	2	0	0	2	[143]
Khung (1966)	2	0	0	0	[65]
Moore (1968)	15	1	9	–	[88]
Rochlin (1962)	3	0	0	0	[108]
FUDR					
Ansfield (1962)	3	1	–	–	[6]
Wilson (1967)	21	1	11	–	[144]
Cytosine arabinoside					
Frei (1969)	2	0	0	–	[36]
G-mercaptopurine					
Regelson (1967)	15	2	0	–	[104]
Lemon (1964)	1	1	0	–	[73][a]

CR, complete response; *PR*, partial response: 50% reduction of the product of the tumor diameters; *MR*, minimal response: < 50% (often 'response' without any indication of magnitude of response); *O*, none; –, not recorded
[a] Case reports

Table 11. Single-agent chemotherapy: Miscellaneous agents

Drug Author (year)	No. of patients	No. of CR & PR	MR/stabi- lization	Subjective response	Reference no.
Hydroxyurea					
Falkson (1967)	1	0	0	1	[28]
Lerner (1965)	1	0	0	–	[74]
Nevinny (1968)	18	5	–	–	[93]
Stolbach (1981)	19	1	3		[121]
Methyl-Gag					
Knight (1979, 1980)	23	3	7		[68, 69]
Todd (1980, 1981)	25	4	9	–	[129, 130]
Zeffren (1981)	31	0	5	–	[148]
Killien (1980)	2	1	–	–	[66]
m-AMSA					
Schneider (1980)	20	1	0	–	[114]
Van Echo (1980)	16	0	4	–	[132]
Dianhydrogalactitol					
Hahn (1979)	35	0	–	–	[45]
Piperazinedione					
Pasmantier (1977)	20	9	–	–	[100]
Mitotane					
Hogan (1981)	12	0	0	–	[51]

CR, complete response; *PR*, partial response: 50% reduction of the product of the tumor diameters; *MR*, minimal response: < 50% (often 'response' without any indication of magnitude of response); *O*, none; –, not recorded

Table 12. Multi-agent chemotherapy in renal cell carcinoma

Author (year)	Drugs	No. of patients	No. of CR & PR	MR/stabi-lization	Subjective response	Reference no.
I. Regimens that include vinblastine						
Davis (1978)	Vinblastine, CCNU	29	7	0	0	[22]
Merrin (1975)	Vinblastine, CCNU	6	1	3	–	[83]
Merrin (1975)	Vinblastine, MeCCNU	15	1	6	–	[83]
Levi (1980)	Vinblastine, bleomycin, HDMTX	14	5	4	–	[75]
Samson (1976)	Vinblastine, bleomycin, cis-platinum	4	0	–	–	[112]
Hahn (1981)	Vinblastine, CCNU	60	3	–	–	[46]
Knost (1981)	Vinblastine, bleomycin	15	2	0	–	[70]
II. Other regimens						
Johnson (1975)	Vincristine + hydroxyurea	15	0	2	0	[60]
Baumgartner (1980)	Vincristine, bleomycin, HDMTX, + (cyclophosphamide or peptochemio)	12	2	5	–	[8]
Dana (1981)	Adriamycin, bleomycin, vincristine, cyclo-phosphamide, BCG	13	3	8		[21]
Werf-Messing (1974)	Cyclophosphamide, 5-fluorouracil, methotrexate, vincristine	18	0	–	1	[141]

CR, complete response; *PR*, partial response: 50% reduction of the product of the tumor diameters; *MR*, minimal response: < 50% (often 'response' without any indication of magnitude of response); *O*, none; –, not recorded

5-Fluorouracil appears to have minimal activity; virtually all of the studies are phase I studies (Table 10). Hydroxyurea showed some activity in early trials. Methyl-glyoxal-bis-guanylhydrazone (methyl-GAG) appeared to have activity, but more recent reports have not been encouraging (Table 11).

Recent studies of agents in renal cell carcinoma have included essentially negative studies of N-[4-(9-acridinyl-amino)-3-methoxyphenyl]-methanesulfonamide (m-AMSA), with one response in 36 evaluable patients in the two series reported [114, 132]. Other negative studies included high-dose cyclophosphamide at 40 mg/m² with 0 of 12 responses, as well as high-dose tamoxifen at 100 mg/m² with none of three responses. Other tamoxifen studies have demonstrated minimal activity (Table 4). Interesting but preliminary reports suggest that adjunctive nephrectomy is an important predictor of response to chemotherapy [56]. A variety of chemotherapeutic agents were studied with responses seen only in those patients who had prior nephrectomy. This study will require careful confirmation.

Chemotherapy has also been used in a recent trial as a true adjuvant to the surgical treatment of hypernephroma. Miller et al. [84] reported in 1980 that a combination of bleomycin and CCNU was an effective adjuvant in 16 patients with stage II or III renal cell carcinomas. Eleven of the 16 patients remained disease-free from 12.7 to 70.4 months with a median disease-free survival of 3.7 years. This study was not randomized. Their conclusion was based on a comparison with historical controls. In this study, two of the patients died of bleomycin pulmonary toxicity.

Combination Chemotherapy

Combination chemotherapy has shown no distinct benefit over single-agent chemotherapy. No randomized trial shows its advantage; occasional studies appear to have higher response rates than when single agents are used alone. Table 12 demonstrates the accumulated literature on combination chemotherapy in hypernephromas. Of interest is the recent combination of vinblastine, high-dose methotrexate, and bleomycin, which was used with or without tamoxifen [75]. There were five PRs in 14 patients for a response rate of 36%, as well as another 10 minimal responses, with less than 50% regression of tumor. The addition of tamoxifen did not appear to affect significantly response rate. In terms of toxicity, 3% of the courses were associated with white blood cell counts of less than 2,000 or platelet counts less than 100,000. Whether this combination of chemotherapy is better than single-agent vinblastine will need to be tested further. Of interest is the use of high-dose methotrexate, which has not been adequately studied in this disease.

References

1. Alberto P, Senn HJ (1974) Hormonal therapy of renal carcinoma alone and in association with cytostatic drugs. Cancer 33: 1226–1229
2. Al-Sarraf M (1979) Abstract: The clinical trial of tamoxifen in patients with advanced renal cell cancer: a Southwest Oncology Group study. Proc AACR ASCO 20: 378
3. Al-Sarraf M, Eyre H, Bonnet J, Saiki J, Gagliano R, Pugh R, Lehane D, Dixon D, Bottomley R (1981) Study of tamoxifen in metastatic renal cell carcinoma and the influence of certain prognostic factors: a southwest oncology group study. Cancer Treat Rep 65: 447–451

4. Anders CJ, Kemp NH (1961) Cyclophosphamide in treatment of disseminated malignant disease. Br Med J 2: 1516–1523

5. Andrews NC, Wilson WL (1967) Phase II study of methotrexate (NSC-740) in solid tumors. Cancer Chemother Rep 51: 471–474

6. Ansfield FJ, Schroeder JM, Curreri AR (1962) A preliminary comparison of 5-fluoro-2′deoxyuridine administered by rapid daily intravenous injections and by slow continuous infusion. Cancer Chemother Rep 16: 289–390

7. Atkins HL, Gregg HG, Hyman GA (1962) Clinical appraisal of cyclophosphamide in malignant neoplasms. Cancer 15: 1076–1080

8. Baumgartner G, Heinz R, Arbes H, Lenzhoffer R, Pridun N, Schuller J (1980) Methotrexate-citrovorum factor used alone and in combination chemotherapy for advanced hypernephromas. Cancer Treat Rep 64: 41–46

9. Baumgartner G, Heinz R, Linemayr G (1980) Methotrexate citrovorum factor therapy in advanced hypernephromas. (Germ) Wien Klin Wochenschr 92(15): 526–530

10. Bergman SM, Lippert M, Javadpour (1980) The value of whole lung tomography in the early detection of metastatic disease in patients with renal cell carcinoma and testicular tumors. J Urol 124: 860–862

11. Bergsagel DE, Levin WC (1960) A prelusive clinical trial of cyclophosphamide. Cancer Chemother Rep 8: 120–134

12. Bloom HJG, Wallace DM (1964) Hormones and the kidney: Possible therapeutic role of testosterone in a patient with regression of metastases from renal adenocarcinoma. Br Med J 2: 476–480

13. Bloom HJG (1971) Medroxyprogesterone acetate (Provera) in the treatment of metastatic renal cancer. Br J Cancer 25: 250–265

14. Bloom HJG (1973) Hormone-induced and spontaneous regression of metastatic renal cancer. Cancer 32: 1066–1071

15. Boxer RJ, Waisman J, Lieber MM, Manpaso FM, Skinner DG (1979) Renal carcinoma: computer analysis of 96 patients treated by nephrectomy. J Urol 122: 598–601

16. Bukowski RM, LoBuglio A, McCracken J, Pugh R (1980) Phase II trial of Baker's antifol in metastatic renal cell carcinoma: A Southwest Oncology Group Study. Cancer Treat Rep 64: 1387–1388

17. Carter SK, Wasserman TH (1975) The chemotherapy of urologic cancer. Cancer 36: 729–747

18. Choy DSJ, Arandia J, Rosenbaum I (1967) Clinical evaluation of a new alkylating agent, azetepa, in one hundred and twenty-five cases of malignant tumors. Int J Cancer 2: 189–193

19. Concolino G, Marocchi A, Conti C, Tenaglia R, Silverio F, Brace U (1978) Human renal cell carcinoma as a hormone-dependent tumor. Cancer Res 38: 4340–4344

20. Costa G, Hreshchyshyn MM, Holland JF (1962) Initial clinical studies with vincristine. Cancer Chemother Rep 24: 39–44

21. Dana BW, Alberts DS (1981) Combination chemoimmunotherapy for advanced renal carcinoma with Adriamycin, bleomycin, vincristine, cyclophosphamide, plug BCG. Cancer Clin Trials 4: 205–207

22. Davis TE, Manalo FB (1978) Combination chemotherapy of advanced renal cell cancer with CCNU and vinblastine. Proc AACR ASCO 19: 316

23. DeKernion JB, Ramming KP, Smith RB (1978) The natural history of metastatic renal cell carcinoma: computer analysis. J Urol 120: 148–152

24. DeKernion JB (1980) Lymphadenectomy for renal cell carcinoma: therapeutic implications. Urol Clin North Am 7: 697

25. Dick DAL, Phillips AF (1961) Clinical experience with cyclophosphamide in malignant disease. Can Med Assoc J 85: 947–986

26. Dorn III W, Gladden MP, Rankin EA (1975) Regression of a renal-cell metastatic osseous lesion following treatment. Bone Joint Surg 57A: 869–870

27. Fairlamb DJ (1981) Spontaneous regression of metastases of renal cancer: a report of two cases including the first recorded regression following irradiation of a dominant metastasis and review of the world literature. Cancer 47: 2102–2106
28. Falkson HC, Falkson G (1967) A clinical trial with hydroxyurea. Med Proc 13: 436–438
29. Ferrazzi E, Salvagno L, Fornasiero A, Cartei G, Fiorentino M (1980) Tamoxifen treatment for advanced renal cell cancer. Tumori 66: 601–605
30. Feun LG, Drelichman A, Singhakowinte A, Vaitkevicius VK (1979) Letters: Phase II study of nafoxidine in the therapy for advanced renal carcinoma. Cancer Treat Rep 63: 149–150
31. Finney R (1973) An evaluation of postoperative radiotherapy in hypernephroma treatment – A clinical trial. Cancer 32: 1332–1340
32. Fossa SD, Talle K (1980) Treatment of metastatic renal cancer with ifosfamide and mesnum with or without irradiation. Cancer Treat Rep 64: 1103–1108
33. Fox MF (1965) The effect of cyclophosphamide on some urinary tract tumors. Br J Urol 37: 399–409
34. Freed SZ, Halperin JP, Gordon M (1977) Idiopathic regression of metastases from renal cell carcinoma. J Urol 118: 538–541
35. Frei III E, Franzino A, Shnider BI, Costa G, Colsky J, Brindley CO, Hosley H, Holland JF, Gold GL, Jonsson U (1961) Clinical studies of vinblastine. Cancer Chemother Rep 12: 125–129
36. Frei III E, Bickers JN, Hewlett JS, Lane M, Leary WV, Talley RW (1969) Dose schedule and antitumor studies of arabinosyl cytosine (NSC 63878). Cancer Res 29: 1325–1332
37. Garfield DH, Kennedy BJ (1972) Regression of metastatic renal cell carcinoma following nephrectomy. Cancer 30: 190–196
38. Glick JH, Wein A, Torri S, Alavi J, Harris D, Brodovsky H (1980) Phase II study of tamoxifen in patients with advanced renal cell carcinoma. Cancer Treat Rep 64: 343–344
39. Gralla RJ, Yagoda A (1979) Phase II evaluation of chlorozotocin in patients with renal cell carcinoma. Cancer Treat Rep 63: 1007–1008
40. Hagan K, Trapp JD, Rhany RK, Reynolds VH (1974) Treatment of metastatic renal cell carcinoma. South Med J 67: 1175–1178
41. Hahn DM, Schimpff S, Wiernik P, Sutherland J (1976) Single agent therapy for hypernephroma: CCNU, vinblastine, thiotepa & bleomycin. Proc AACR ASCO 17: 82
42. Hahn DM, Schimpff SC (1977) Single-agent therapy for renal cell carcinoma: CCNU, vinblastine, thioTEPA, or bleomycin. Cancer Treat Rep 61: 1585–1587
43. Hahn RG, Brodovsky H (1976) Abstract: Methyl CCNU, velban and depo-provera treatment trials in advanced renal cancer. Proc AACR ASCO 17: 246
44. Hahn RG, Temkin NR, Savlov ED, Perlia C, Wampler GL, Horton J, Marsh J, Carbone PP (1978) Phase II Study of vinblastine, methyl-CCNU, and medroxyprogesterone in advanced renal cell cancer. Cancer Treat Rep 62: 1093–1095
45. Hahn RG, Bauer M, Wolter J, Creech R, Bennett JM, Wampler GL (1979) Phase II Study of single-agent therapy with megestrol acetate, VP-16–213, cyclophosphamide, and dianhydrogalactitol in advanced renal cell cancer. Cancer Treat Rep 63: 513–515
46. Hahn RG, Begg CB, Davis T (1981) Phase II study of vinblastine-CCNU, triazinate, and dactinomycin in advanced renal cell cancer. Cancer Treat Rep 65: 711–713
47. Haskell CM, Ossorio RC (1976) Abstract: Chemoimmunotherapy of metastatic breast cancer with Corynebacterium parvum (CP): A double blind randomized trial. Proc AACR ASCO 17: 265
48. Hill JM, Loeb E (1961) Treatment of leukemia, lymphoma, and other malignant neoplasms with vinblastine. Cancer Chemother Rep 15: 41–61
49. Hindmarsh JR, Hall RR, Kulatilake AE (1979) Renal cell carcinoma: A preliminary clinical trial of methodichlorophen (D.D.M.P.). Clin Oncol 5: 11–15

50. Hire EA, Samson MK (1979) Use of VM-26 as a single agent in the treatment of renal carcinoma. Cancer Clin Trials 2:293–295

51. Hogan TF, Citrin DL, Freeberg BL (1981) A preliminary report of mitotane therapy of advanced renal and prostate cancer. Cancer Treat Rep 65:539–540

52. Hogan TF (1979) Hormonal Therapy of Renal-Cell Carcinoma. In: Rose DP (ed) Endocrinology of Cancer. CRC, Boca Raton, pp 70–86

53. Horn Y, Hochman A (1967) The alkaloids of vinca rosea linn in malignant tumors. Oncology 21:214–220

54. Hrushesky WJ, Murphy GP (1977) Current status of the therapy of advanced renal carcinoma. J Surg Oncol 9:277–288

55. Hrushesky WJ (1977) Abstract: What's old and new in advanced renal cell carcinoma. Proc AACR ASCO 18:318

56. Ishmael DR, Bottomley R, Geyer J (1980) Effect of nephrectomy on eventual response to chemotherapy in renal cell carcinoma. Proc AACR ASCO 21:429

57. Ishmael DR, Burpo LJ, Bottomley RH (1978) Abstract: Combined therapy of advanced hypernephroma with medroxyprogesterone, BCG, Adriamycin and vincristine. Proc AACR ASCO 19:407

58. Jenkin RDT (1967) Correspondence: Androgens in metastatic renal adenocarcinoma. Br Med J 11:361

59. Johnson DE, Kaesler KE, Samuels ML (1975) Is nephrectomy justified in patients with metastatic renal cell carcinoma. J Urol 114:27

60. Johnson DE, Rodriguez L, Holoye PY, Samuels ML (1975) Combination vincristine (NSC-67574) and hydroxyurea (NSC-32065) for metastatic renal carcinoma. Cancer Chemother Rep 59:1159–1160

61. Johnson DE, Chalbaud RA, Holoye PY, Samuels ML (1975) Clinical trial of bleomycin (NSC-125066) in the treatment of metastatic renal carcinoma. Cancer Chemother Rep 59:433–435

62. Juusela H, Malmio K, Alfthan O, Oravisto KJ (1977) Preoperative irradiation in the treatment of renal adenocarcinoma. Scand J Urol Nephrol 11:277

63. Katakkar SB, Franks CR (1978) Chemo-hormonal therapy for metastatic renal cell carcinoma with Adriamycin, hydroxyurea, vinblastine, and medroxyprogesterone acetate. Cancer Treat Rep 62:1379–1380

64. Kato T, Nemoto R, Mori H, Kumagai I (1979) Correspondence: Microencapsulated mitomycin-C therapy in renal-cell carcinoma. Lancet 1:479–480

65. Khung CL, Hall TC, Piro AJ, Dederick MM (1966) A clinical trial of oral 5-fluorouracil. Clin Pharmacol Ther 7:527–533

66. Killien J, Hoth D, Smith F, Schein P, Woolley P, Lombardi VT (1980) Methyl-glyoxal-bis-quanylhydrazone (NSC 32946) (Methyl-G): Phase II experience and clinical pharmacology. Proc AACR ASCO 21:368

67. Kiruluta G, Morales A, Lott S (1975) Response of renal adenocarcinoma to cyclophosphamide. Urology 6:557–558

68. Knight WA, Livingston RB, Fabian D, Costanzi J (1979) Phase I-II trial of methly-GAG: A southwest oncology group pilot study. Cancer Treat Rep 63:1933–1937

69. Knight WA, Livingston RB, Fabian C, Costanzi J (1980) Methylglyoxal-bis-guanylhydrazone (methyl GAG, MGBG) in advanced renal carcinoma. Proc AACR ASCO 21:367

70. Knost JA, Oldham RK, Hande KR, Rhamy RK, Greco FA (1981) Combination of vinblastine and bleomycin in metastatic renal cell carcinoma. Cancer Treat Rep 65:349–350

71. Kofman S, Eisenstein R (1963) Mithramycin in the treatment of disseminated cancer. Cancer Chemother Rep 32:77–96

72. Legha S, Muggia FM (1976) Antiestrogens in the treatment of cancer (correspondence). Ann Intern Med 84:751

73. Lemon HM, Miller DM, Smith J, Walker EE (1964) Remission of metastases of erythropoietin-secreting renal cell adenocarcinoma after 6-mercaptopurine (NSC-755) therapy. Cancer Chemother Rep 36: 49–140

74. Lerner H, Beckloff GL (1965) Hydroxyurea administered intermittently JAMA 192: 138–140

75. Levi JA, Dalley D, Aroney R (1980) Abstract: A comparative trial of the combination vinblastine (V), methotrexate (A) and bleomycin (B) with and without tamoxifen (T) for metastatic renal cell carcinoma (RCC). Proc AACR ASCO 21: 426

76. Lokich JJ, Harrison JH (1975) Renal cell carcinoma: Natural history and chemotherapeutic experience. J Urol 114: 371–374

77. Love DR (1979) Computed tomograph staging of renal carcinoma. Urol Radiol 1: 3

78. Luce JK, Thurman WG, Issacs BL, Talley RW (1970) Clinical trials with the antitumor agent 5-(3,3-dimethyl-1-triazeno)imidazole-4-carboxamide (NSC-45388). Cancer Chemother Rep 54: 119–124

79. MacErlean DP, Owena AP, Bryan PJ (1980) Hypernephroma embolisation – is it worthwhile? Clin Radiol 31: 297–300

80. Maskens AP, Hap B, Kozyreff VN, Callewaert W, Lion G, Van den Abbeele KG (1980) Abstract: Serum levels of medroxyprogesterone acetate under various treatment schedules. Proc AACR ASCO 21: 165

81. McNichols DW, Segura JW, Wu S, Safire GE (1981) Renal cell carcinoma: Long-term survival and late recurrence. J Urol 126: 17–23

82. Melander O, Notter G, Schreeb T von (1967) Hormone treatment of metastasizing renal cancer. Nord Med 78: 1309

83. Merrin C, Mittleman A, Fanous N, Wajsman Z, Murphy GP (1975) Chemotherapy of advanced renal cell carcinoma with vinblastine and CCNU. J Urol 113: 21–23

84. Miller CF, Blom J, Tripler AMC, Reed N (1980) Abstract: Adjuvant chemotherapy of renal cell carcinoma using a combination of bleomycin (BLM) and lomustine (CCNU). Proc AACR ASCO 21: 362

85. Mittelman A, Albert DJ, Murphy GP (1973) Lomustine treatment of metastatic renal cell carcinoma. JAMA 225: 32–35

86. Montie JE, Stewart BH, Straffon RA, Banowsky LHW, Hewitt CB, Montague DK (1977) The role of adjunctive nephrectomy in patients with metastatic renal cell carcinoma. J Urol 117: 272–275

87. Moore GE, Brass DJ, Ausman R, Nadler S, Jones R, Slack N, Rimm AA (1968) Effects of chlorambucil (NSC-3088) in 374 patients with advanced cancer. Cancer Chemother Rep 52: 661–666

88. Moore GE, Brass DJ, Audman R, Nadler S, Jones R, Slack N, Rimm AA (1968) Effects of 5-fluorouracil (NSC-19893) in 389 patients with cancer. Cancer Chemother Rep 52: 641–653

89. Morales A, Kiruluta G, Lott S (1975) Hormones in the treatment of metastatic renal cancer. J Urol 114: 692–693

90. Morales A, Wilson JL, Pater JL, Loeb M (1982) Cyto-reductive surgery and systemic bacillus Calmette-guerin therapy in metastatic renal cancer: A phase II trial. J Urol 127: 230–235

91. Mulder JH, Alexieva-Figusch I (1979) Abstract: Tamoxifen in metastatic renal cell carcinoma (meeting abstract). Cancer Treat Rep 63(7): 1222

92. Murphy GP (1978) Chemotherapy of renal, bladder, and prostate cancer. In: Brodsky I, Kahn SB, Conroy J (eds) Cancer chemotherapy III. Grune & Stratton, New York, pp 179–194

93. Nevinny HB, Hall TC (1968) Chemotherapy with hydroxyurea (NSC-32065) in renal cell carcinoma. J Clin Pharmacol 8: 352–359

94. O'Bryan RM, Luce JK, Talley RW, Gottlieb JA, Baker LH, Bonadonna G (1973) Phase II evaluation of Adriamycin in human neoplasia. Cancer 32: 1–8

95. O'Dea MJ, Zincke H, Utz DC, Bernatz PE (1978) The treatment of renal cell carcinoma with solitary metastasis. J Urol 120:540–542

96. Paine CH, Wright FW, Ellis F (1970) The use of progestogen in the treatment of metastatic carcinoma of the kidney and uterine body. Br J Cancer 24:277–282

97. Paladine W, Longacre D, Hemmings P, Harper G (1979) Nafoxidine, an antiestrogen in hypernephroma (ASCO abs). Proc AACR ASCO 20:293

98. Papac R, Luikhart S, Kirkwood J (1980) Abstract: High dose tamoxifen in patients with advanced renal cell cancer and malignant melanoma. Proc AACR ASCO 20:358

99. Papac RJ, Ross SA, Levy A (1977) Renal cell carcinoma: Analysis of 31 cases with assessment of endocrine therapy. Am J Med Sci 274:281–290

100. Pasmantier MW, Coleman M, Kennedy BJ, Eagan R, Carolla R, Weiss R, Leone L, Silver RT (1977) Piperazinedione in metastatic renal papac carcinoma. Cancer Treat Rep 61:1731–1732

101. Patel NP, Lavengood RW (1978) Renal cell carcinoma: Natural history and results of treatment. J Urol 119:722–726

102. Peterson LJ, Grimes JH, Dees JE, Anderson EE (1974) Hormonal therapy in metastatic hypernephroma. Urology 4:669–673

103. Ramirez G, Weiss AJ, Rochlin DB, Bisel HF (1971) Phase II study of 6-methyl-pregn-r-ene-3,11,20-trione (NSC-17256). Cancer Chemother Rep 55:265–268

104. Regelson W, Holland JF, Gold GL, Lynch J, Olson KB, Horton J, Hall TC, Krant M, Colsky J, Miller SP, Owens A (1967) 6-mercaptopurine (NSC-755) given intravenously at weekly intervals to patients with advanced cancer. Cancer Chemother Rep 51:277–282

105. Richards II Frederick, Muss HB, White DR, Cooper MR, Spurr CL (1977) CCNU, bleomycin, and methylprednisolone with or without Adriamycin in renal cell carcinoma: A randomized trial. Cancer Treat Rep 61:1591–1593

106. Richie JP, Wand BS, Steele GD, Wilson RE, Mannick JA (1980) In vivo and in vitro effects of xenogeneic immune ribonucleic acid in patients with advanced renal cell carcinoma: A phase I study. J Urol 126:24–28

107. Robson CJ, Churchill BM, Anderson W (1969) The results of radical nephrectomy for renal cell carcinoma. J Urol 101:297–301

108. Rochlin DB, Shiner J, Langdon E, Ottoman R (1962) Use of 5-fluorouracil in disseminated solid neoplasms. Ann Surg 156:105–113

109. Rodriguez LH, Johnson DE (1978) Clinical trial of cis-platinum (NSC 119875) in metastatic renal cell carcinoma. Urology 11:344–346

110. Sadoff L, Lusk W (1974) The effect of large doses of medroxyprogesterone acetate (MPA) on urinary estrogen levels and serum levels of cortisol T^4 LH and testosterone in patients with advanced cancer. Obstet Gynecol 43:262–267

111. Salimtschik M, Mouridsen HT, Loeber J, Johansson E (1980) Comparative pharmaco-kinetics of medroxyprogesterone acetate administered by oral and intramuscular routes. Cancer Chemother Pharmacol 4:267–269

112. Samson MK, Baker LH, Devos JM, Burker TR, Izbicki RM, Vaitkevicius VK (1976) Phase I clinical trial of combined therapy with vinblastine (NSC-49842), bleomycin (NSC-125066), and cis-dichlorodiammineplatinum(II) (NSC-119875). Cancer Treat Rep 60:91–97

113. Samuels ML, Sullivan P, Howe GD (1968) Medroxyprogesterone acetate in the treatment of renal cell carcinoma (hypernephroma). Cancer 22:525–532

114. Schneider RJ, Woodcock TM, Yagoda A (1980) Phase II trial of 4'-(9-acridinylami-no)methanesulfon-m-anisidide (AMSA) in patients with metastatic hypernephroma. Cancer Treat Rep 64:183–185

115. Schumacher HR, O'Connell JP (1963) The intravenous use of uracil mustard (U-8344). Cancer 16:345–349

116. Shnider BI, Gold GL, Hall T, Dederick M, Nevinny HB, Patee KG, Lasagna L, Owens AH, Hreschyshyn M, Selawry O, Holland JF, Franzino A, Zubrod CG, Frei E, Brindley C (1960) Preliminary studies with cyclophosphamide. Cancer Chemother Rep 8:106–111

117. Skinner DG, Colvin RB, Vermillion CD, Pfister RC, Leadbetter WF (1971) Diagnosis and management of renal cell carcinoma. A clinical and pathologic study of 309 cases. Cancer 28: 1165−1177
118. Skinner DG, DeKernion JG (eds) (1978) Genitourinary Cancer, Saunders, Philadelphia, pp 128−129
119. Smart CR, Rochlin DB, Nahum AM, Silva A, Wagner D (1964) Clinical experience with vinblastine sulfate (NSC-49842) in squamous cell carcinoma and other malignancies. Cancer Chemother Rep 34: 31−45
120. Solomon J, Alexander MJ, Steinfeld J (1963) Cyclophosphamide: a clinical study. JAMA 183: 165−170
121. Stolbach LL, Begg CB, Hall T, Horton J (1981) Treatment of renal carcinoma: A phase III randomized trial of oral medroxyprogesterone (Provera), hydroxyurea, and nafoxidine. Cancer Treat Rep 65: 689−692
122. Swanson DA, Johnson DE (1980) A clinical trial of estramustine phosphate (NSC 89199) in the management of metastatic renal cell carcinoma (meeting abstract). Proc AACR ASCO 21: 346
123. Swanson DA, Johnson DE (1981) Estramustine phosphate (EMCYT) as treatment for metastatic renal carcinoma. Urology 17: 344−346
124. Swanson DA, Wallace S, Johnson DE (1980) The role of embolization and nephrectomy in the treatment of metastatic renal carcinoma. Urol Clin North Am 7: 719−730
124. Talley RW (1973) Chemotherapy of the adenocarcinoma of the kidney. Cancer 32: 1062−1065
126. Talley RW, Moorhead EL, Tucker WG, SanDiego EL, Brennan MJ (1969) Treatment of metastatic hypernephroma. JAMA 207: 322−328
127. Talley RW, Oberhauser NA, Brownlee RW, O'Bryan RM (1979) Chemotherapy of metastatic renal adenocarcinoma with a five-drug regimen. Henry Ford Hosp Med J 27: 110−112
128. Tisman G, Kellon DB, Wu S, Safire GE (1976) Use of tamoxifen in tumors other than breast cancer. Clin Res 24: 381A
129. Todd III RF, Garnick MB, Canellos GP (1980) Abstract: Chemotherapy of advanced renal adenocarcinoma with methyl-glyoxal-BIS-guanylhydrazone (methyl-GAG). Proc AACR ASCO 21: 340
130. Todd FR, Garnick MB, Canellos GP, Richie JP, Gittes RF, Mayer RJ, Skarin AT (1981) Phase I-II trial of methyl-GAG in the treatment of patients with metastatic renal adenocarcinoma. Cancer Treat Rep 65: 17−20
131. Tolia BM, Whitmore WF Jr (1975) Solitary metastasis from renal cell carcinoma. J Urol 114: 836−837
132. Van Echo DA, Markus S, Aisner J, Wiernik PH (1980) Phase II trial of 4′-(9-acri-dinylamino)methanesulfon-m-anisidide (AMSA) in patients with metastatic renal cell carcinoma. Cancer Treat Rep 64: 1009−1010
133. Vosika GJ, Ryan MJ, Fortuny IA, Meyer C, Kiang DT, Theologides A, Kennedy BJ (1978) CCNU vinblastine and delalutin therapy in renal cell carcinoma. Med Pediatr Oncol 5: 89−91
134. Wagle DG, Murphy GP (1971) Hormonal therapy in advanced renal cell carcinoma. Cancer 28: 318−321
135. Wajsman Z, Beckley S, Madajewicz S, Dragone N (1980) Abstract: high dose cyclophosphamide (CPM) in metastatic renal cell cancer. Proc AACR ASCO 21: 423
136. Watne AL, Badillo J, Koike A, Kondo T, Moore GE (1960) Clinical studies of actinomycin D. Ann NY Acad Sci 89: 445−453
137. Watne AL, Moore D, Gorgun B (1967) Solid tumor chemotherapy with mitomycin C. Arch Surg 95: 175−178

138. Weiselberg L, Budman D, Vinciguerra V, Schulman P, Degnan TJ (1981) Tamoxifen in unresectable hypernephroma: A phase II trial and review of the literature. Cancer Clin Trials 4: 195–198
139. Weiss AJ, Jackson LG, Carabasi R (1961) An evaluation of 5-fluorouracil in malignant disease. Ann Intern Med 55: 731–741
140. Werf-Messing B Van der (1973) Carcinoma of the kidney. Cancer 32: 1056–1066
141. Werf-Messing B Van der, Mulder J (1974) Metastatic kidney cancer treated with multiple drug therapy at the Rotterdam Radiotherapy Institute. Br J Cancer 29: 491–492
142. Werf-Messing B Van der, Van Gilse HA (1971) Hormonal treatment of metastases of renal carcinoma. Br J Cancer 25: 423–427
143. White JE, Ricketts WN, Strudwick WJ (1962) A clinical study of 5-fluorouracil in a variety of far advanced human malignancies. J Natl Med Assoc 54: 315
144. Wilson WL, Bisel HF, Krementa ET, Lein RC, Prohaska JV (1967) Further clinical evaluation of 2'-deoxy-5-fluorouridine (NSC-27640). Cancer Chemother Rep 51: 85–90
145. Wong PP, Yagoda A, Currie VE, Young CA (1977) Phase II study of vindesine sulfate in the therapy for advanced renal carcinoma. Cancer Treat Rep 61: 1727–1729
146. Woodruff MW, Wagle D, Gailani SD, Jones R (1967) The current status of chemotherapy for advanced renal carcinoma. J Urol 97: 611–618
147. Wright TL, Hurley J, Korst DR, Monto RW, Rohn RJ, Will JJ, Louis J (1963) Vinblastine in neoplastic disease. Cancer Res 23: 169–179
148. Zeffren J, Yagoda A, Watson RC, Natale RB, Blumenreich MS, Chapman R, Howard J (1981) Phase II trial of methyl-GAG in advanced renal cancer. Cancer Treat Rep 65: 525–527

Penile Cancer Chemotherapy

F. J. Meyers

Division of Hematology/Oncology, University of California, Davis Medical Center, Sacramento, CA, USA

Introduction

Penile cancer has attracted little attention because of its rarity in the USA and Europe. However, in certain countries of Africa (e.g., Uganda), and Asia (e.g., Japan), and North America (e.g., Puerto Rico, Mexico), it is quite common [15]. Thus, a current knowledge of the therapy of penile carcinoma is important in order to provide optimal care to this large group of people and to formulate clinical trials that will improve care.

Spread

The lymphatics of the penile shaft and prepuce converge at the base of the penis and then separate to terminate in the superficial inguinal nodes. Anastamoses between each side allow unilateral lesions of the penis to drain contralaterally. Secondary drainage is to the pelvic lymph nodes. The glans and the urethra drain directly to the pelvic nodes.

Staging

Two systems have been used to stage penile carcinoma (Table 1).
The presence or absence of lymph node involvement is critical in assigning prognosis [12, 15]. Only 30% of patients with positive nodes will survive 5 years in contrast to 80% with negative nodes (normal estimated survival for age). However, clinical staging of the inguinal nodes is frequently inaccurate. Infection of the primary tumor with resultant reactive adenopathy leads to 30%−65% of palpable nodes being free of tumor [2, 15]. Similarly, tumor involvement in nonpalpable nodes is approximately 20%. Thus, considerable controversy exists over the management of the inguinal nodes [1, 6]. In the absence of obviously malignant nodes, a 6 week healing period after primary therapy is recommended. If nodes remain palpable, a node dissection can be done without compromising survival rates.

Treatment

Simple circumcision is sometimes used for small lesions confined to the prepuce. Partial penectomy is the standard therapy for most primary lesions involving the distal

Recent Results in Cancer Research. Vol. 85
© Springer-Verlag Berlin · Heidelberg 1983

Table 1. Comparison of the two most frequently used staging systems

	Jackson stage [10]	UICC T, N, M [21]
I	Tumor limited to the glans or prepuce	
	Tumor 2 cm or less in largest dimension, superficial	T_1, N_0, M_0
	Tumor greater than 2 cm, less than 5 cm, minimal infiltration	T_2, N_0, M_0
II	Invasion into the shaft or corpora without nodal metastases	
	Tumor greater than 5 cm or any size with deep infiltration	T_3, N_0, M_0
III	Confined to the shaft but with mobile inguinal node involvement	
	Unilateral	Any T, N_1, M_0
	Bilateral	Any T, N_2, M_0
IV	Local invasion beyond the shaft	T_4
	Inoperable or juxtaregional lymph node metastases	Any T, N_3, or N_4, M_0
	Distant metastases	Any T, any N, M_1

penis [8, 12, 18]. However, excellent local control rates using radiation therapy with preservation of sexual function and micturition have been reported [7, 11, 17]. Unfortunately, there are no randomized trials with comparable patients that define guidelines for choosing one or the other therapy.

Chemotherapy

Drug therapy has been employed for all stages of penile carcinoma. As with surgery and radiation, the paucity of carefully done clinical trials has impeded confident definition of the role of chemotherapy in this disease. Enough data exists, however, to propose treatment guidelines and to prepare the way for future trials.

The Primary Lesion — Drug Therapy Alone

Bleomycin has been used in the treatment of the primary tumor by five different groups and all five report a response rate, complete and partial, of 50%–70%. Rathert and Lutzeyer reported three complete responses among six evaluable patients [16]. One patient had recurrent disease at 2 months and subsequently received radiation and surgery. The two other patients had simple circumcision following chemotherapy and were free of disease 2 and 3 years later. These three patients received a total dose of bleomycin of 300–435 mg.

Folke reported that two of three patients responded to bleomycin [4]. One patient was alive without recurrent disease at 4 years without additional therapy. The other responder (partial response with 90% regression) died of pulmonary fibrosis after receiving 600 mg bleomycin.

Kyalwazi et al. treated 15 patients [13]. Three complete responders were reported; one cancer in situ, one stage I, and one stage II. The patient with stage I disease died after 3 months of unknown cause. The other two patients received no additional therapy; survival and duration of follow-up is not noted. Six patients had partial responses and were continued on drug therapy or had partial amputations. Therefore, 9 of 15 patients had excellent responses to bleomycin.

Ichikawa summarized the experience of 40 institutions in Japan [9]. Twenty-four patients were treated with bleomycin alone. Twelve were alive at last report, six for more than 3 years.

The EORTC reported one patient who achieved a complete response with 420 mg bleomycin [3]. The duration of the response was not noted.

Bleomycin alone has been shown to have significant activity and, used alone, a number of long-term survivals have been achieved. This set the stage for combination therapy of the primary tumor.

Combination Therapy Including Bleomycin for the Primary Lesion

Two series are noteworthy. Ichikawa reviewed the experience at 40 institutions with 164 patients in whom bleomycin was combined with surgery and/or radiation [9]. Of the 164 patients, 123 were alive at the time of the report. In those patients followed for 2 or more years, 60 of 70 were alive. No staging information, drug-dose, or response rate is provided.

Folke reported on seven patients with T_1, T_2, or T_3 lesions (all N_0) who received bleomycin at a dose of 15 mg daily for 5 days every other week during a 5-week course of radiation therapy (4,500 rad) [4]. Six of seven patients had complete responses, three of which were proven by biopsy. One patient had a remnant of tumor excised following the combined therapy. At least two patients had sexual function preserved and all patients maintained normal micturition. No report is available since 1976 that allows ascertainment of 2-year survival.

Single-Agent Drug Therapy of Metastatic Disease

Remarkably, no trials have been published using bleomycin as a single agent for metastatic disease.

Sklaroff and Yagoda treated 11 patients with cis-platinum (CDDP) alone [19]. All had measurable metastatic disease. Six had received prior radiation and eight had received prior chemotherapy (bleomycin-4, methotrexate-5). Nine patients were evaluable for response. Three responders (33%) were noted — one complete response and two partial responses. No dose-response relationship was noted.

These authors also treated eight patients with methotrexate [20]. Five patients received high-dose methotrexate ($250-1,500$ mg/m^2) with citrovorum rescue weekly and three received $0.5-3$ mg/kg weekly. All eight had measurable disease. Three had prior radiation, two had prior bleomycin treatment. Three partial remissions (2/5 high dose, 1/3 low dose) were obtained which lasted 11, 3, and 2 months, respectively. Garnick et al. reported a single patient with multiple subcutaneous and dermal metastases who achieved a clinical complete response after receiving methotrexate 3g/m^2 with citrovorum rescue every week × 10 then every other week × 15 [5]. He died of pneumonitis 9 months after initiation of therapy. A postmortem examination revealed two microscopic tumorous foci.

Combination Chemotherapy

Williams and Blackard treated three patients with vincristine (0.025 mg/kg weekly) and bleomycin (15 mg twice weekly) without observing a response [22]. Lokich and Frie reported a single patient with a partial response to bleomycin and methotrexate [14].

Recommendations

Bleomycin is the most studied and perhaps the most active drug in penile cancer. Whether methotrexate or cis-platinum would have as high a response rate if used against the primary lesion is unknown. Experience with combination chemotherapy is very limited.

Future Prospects

The following approaches would greatly amplify our ability to define the most effective treatment for this disease: (1) A comparison of surgery to radiation with or without bleomycin in the therapy of the primary lesion; (2) an expansion of the data with bleomycin, methotrexate, and cis-platinum as single agents in the treatment of the primary as well as metastatic disease; (3) determination of new active agents; (4) a series of randomized trials of adjuvant chemotherapy in patients with biopsy-proven inguinal node involvement.

No single institution sees the large number of patients necessary to conduct these studies. A national study, as in the testicular intergroup study, or a WHO-sponsored study would be necessary to approach these problems.

References

1. Catalona WJ (1980) Role of lymphadenectomy in carcinoma of the penis. Urol Clin North Am 7: 785–792
2. Droller MJ (1980) Carcinoma of the penis: an overview. Urol Clin North Am 78: 783–784
3. EORTC: Clinical Screening Co-operative Group (1970) Studies of the clinical efficiency of bleomycin in human cancer. Br Med J 2: 643–645
4. Folke, E (1976) Combined treatment with bleomycin in penile carcinomas. GANN Monograph on Cancer Research 19: 231–233
5. Garnick MB, Skarin AT, Steele GA (1979) Metastatic carcinoma of the penis: complete remission after high dose methotrexate chemotherapy. J Urol 122: 265–266
6. Grabstald H (1980) Controversies concerning lymph node dissection for cancer of the penis. Urol Clin North Am 7: 793–799
7. Haile K, Delclos L (1980) The place of radiation therapy in the treatment of carcinoma of the distal end of the penis. Cancer 45: 1980–1984

8. Hanash K, Furlow WL, Utz DC, Harrison EG (1970) Carcinoma of the penis: a clinico pathologic study. J Urol 1094: 291–297
9. Ichikawa T (1977) Chemotherapy of penis carcinoma. In: Grundmann E, Vahlensieck W (eds) Tumors of the male genital system. Springer, Berlin Heidelberg New York, pp 140–156 (Recent results in cancer research, vol 60)
10. Jackson SM (1966) The treatment of carcinoma of the penis. Br J Surg 53: 33–35
11. Kreig RM, Luk KH (1981) Carcinoma of penis: review of cases treated by surgery and radiation therapy 1960–1977. Urology 18: 149–154
12. Kuruvilla JT, Garlick FH, Mammen KE (1971) Results of surgical treatment of carcinoma of the penis. Aust New NZ J Surg 41: 157–159
13. Kyalwazi SK, Bhana D, Harrison NW (1974) Carcinoma of the penis and bleomycin chemotherapy in Uganda. Br J Urol 46: 689–696
14. Lokich JJ, Frei E III (1974) Phase II study of concurrent methotrexate and bleomycin chemotherapy. Cancer Res 34: 2240–2242
15. Persky L (1977) Epidemiology of cancer of the penis. In: Grundmann E, Vahlensieck W (eds) Tumors of the male genital system. Springer Berlin Heidelberg New York, pp 97–109 (Recent results in cancer research, vol 60)
16. Rathert P, Lutzeyer W (1976) Bleomycin effects on malignant tumors of the male genitalia. Prog Biochem Pharmacol 11: 223–230
17. Salaverria JC, Hope-Stone HF, Paris AM, Molland EA, Blandy JP (1979) Conservative treatment of carcinoma of the penis. Br J Urol 51: 32–37
18. Skinner Donald G, Leadbetter W, Kelley S (1972) The surgical management of squamous cell carcinoma of the penis. J Urol 107: 273–277
19. Sklaroff RB, Yagoda A (1979) Cis-diamminedichloride platinum II (DDP) in the treatment of penile carcinoma. Cancer 44: 1563–1565
20. Sklaroff RB, Yagoda A (1980) Methotrexate in the treatment of penile carcinoma. Cancer 45: 214–216
21. UICC (1968) Clinical trials 9: 72
22. Williams R, Blackard CE (1974) Chemotherapy for metastatic squamous cell carcinoma of penis; combination of vincristine and bleomycin. Urology 4: 69–72

Recent Results in Cancer Research

Sponsored by the Swiss League against Cancer. Editor in Chief: P. Rentchnick, Genève

For information about Vols. 1–9, please contact your bookseller of Springer-Verlag